Ultimate Carnivore Diet

THE COMPLETE GUIDE TO LOSING
WEIGHT BY EATING MEAT

RAGNAR ERIKSEN

Ultimate Carnivore Diet   Ragnar Eriksen

ULTIMATE CARNIVORE DIET

Copyright © 2018 by BadCreative
Art Direction, Cover Design & Typography: Gestvlt

ISBN 9781708857813

All rights reserved.
No part of this book may be reproduced or transmitted in any form or by any means, electronic or mechanical, including photocopying, recording, or by any information storage and retrieval system, without permission in writing from the publisher.

This edition contains the complete text

of the original hardcover edition.
NOT ONE WORD HAS BEEN OMITTED.

A Bad Creative Book / published by
arrangement with the author

BAD CREATIVE PUBLISHING HISTORY
Skin Alchemy September 2019
The Simplest Way To Learn Spanish, published March 2017

UPCOMING WORKS

Skin Alchemy For Men, 2020
Skin Alchemy For Teens, 2020

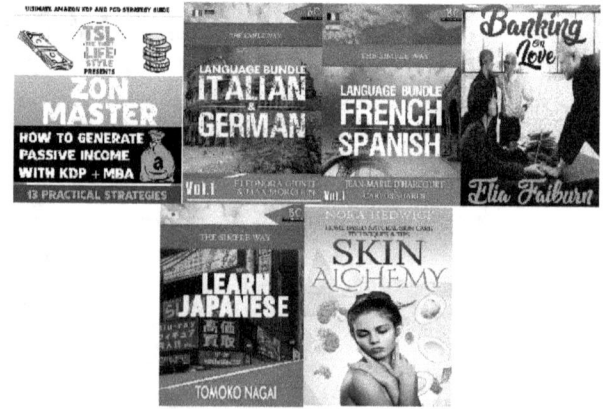

Table of Contents

Introduction 5
Chapter 1 – What This Diet is All About 7
Chapter 2 – Understanding Meat 16
Chapter 3 – Different Ways to Cut Meat 21
Chapter 4 – Seasoning Meat 24
Chapter 5 – Different Methods of Cooking Meat ... 26
Chapter 5 – Carnivore Recipes 30
Chapter 6 – Sample Workout/Meal Plan 94
Chapter 7 – Commonly Asked Questions 101
Conclusion 105

Disclaimer: We are not in the health profession. This outline is what we have used for the past decade or so after many years of changes (iterations) to our diets. If you find additional items to layer in that don't consume a lot of your time feel free to run with it!

Introduction

The Carnivore Diet stems from the belief that humanity's ancestral inhabitants consumed mostly fish and meat, and that the existence of a high carb diet is the main culprit behind many different kinds of chronic diseases.

The truth is, if you're not on a diet with enough meat, eggs and fish, you're probably missing out on a critical nutrient. This nutrient which is essential for brain function and optimal brain development, can also be very important for cardiovascular health. Perhaps most relevant for the modern day, is the fact that a deficiency of it can lead to a non-alcoholic fatty liver (NAFL), which is highly prevalent and associated with diabetes.

The nutrient in question is called choline, and the greatest concentrations of it are found in animal foods.

Unfortunately, today's mainstream dietary advice tends to tether around the mantra "avoid meat and eggs", and is in my opinion, misinformed and malevolent even. I say this because plant-based or vegan diets are wholly inadequate in choline.

The three largest sources of choline are beef liver, eggs, and… human milk. So, by extension, if someone were to be pregnant, or nursing, while getting inadequate choline thanks to the aforementioned diet, it could literally harm the infant's brain development. Some or even most of the epidemic of fatty liver could be down to people avoiding meat and especially, eggs. I highly doubt that nature would have put so much choline in human milk if it weren't so important.

In the recent past, none of this would be happening.

People weren't so easily convinced into thinking that plants are the healthiest foods, or that you shouldn't eat animal foods.

But people have been bamboozled.

The world has gone crazy – nutritionally speaking, and so the lessons to be learned here in this book are simple:

You absolutely need to include animal foods, such as meat, eggs, fish, and dairy in your diet to get adequate choline.

And also, getting good nutrition is equally important for fat loss itself, since when you're well-nourished, you're simply less hungry.

To a large extent, this book is written for meat lovers, and by extension, anyone who wishes to get to know more about this diet, and the many recipes you can prepare on your own. It will give you an overview of the carnivore diet. It will inform you about meat itself, how to cut it, how to season it, how to cook it. It will also debunk some of the ongoing myths that surround the diet and provide you with a 7-day meal plan and workout routine, to help you get started on your journey to weight loss. It's a whole lot of value packed in one place. So, thanks again for getting this book. I hope you enjoy it.

Chapter 1 – What This Diet is All About

The carnivore diet is an all meat-based diet where you completely avoid fruits, vegetables, legumes, grains, nuts, and seeds. It is particularly restrictive in the sense that you are only allowed to eat meat, fish, and other animal byproducts such as eggs and dairy.
Following this diet would require eliminating plant-based food from your diet and in order to get the required dose of energy for the day, advocates of said diet recommend consuming fatty meat cuts. These include beef, lamb, chicken, organ meats, pork, sardines, white fish, turkey, salmon, and just moderate amounts of hard cheese and heavy cream. Bone marrow, lard, and butter are also acceptable.
When it comes to beverages, this diet discourages the drinking of coffee, tea, and other beverages made of plants. You are instead encouraged to have bone broth and water. There is no specificity in caloric requirements per day, or for the amount of meat consumed, and even as to serving sizes. Many proponents of the carnivore diet suggest consuming meat as often as you please, which really won't be often, because the rule of thumb is to eat till you are satiated. This works out in your favor because if you are kept feeling full with proteins, which are the building blocks of muscle, then there is no need for excessive carbs consumption, which are the building blocks of fat, when unchecked via exercise.

There are basically three ways to approach this diet, and they are:
1. Pure Carnivore – this includes consumption of purely animal meat, its fats, NO dairy or animal by-products and water. It's that straightforward and simple.
2. Carnivore – this includes consumption of animal meat, its fat, dairy or animal by-products, and water.

3.   Mostly Carnivore – this includes consumption of animal meat, its fats, dairy or animal by-products, water, and some occasional plant-based food.

Transitioning to this kind of diet is not that challenging. Afterall, many people still opt for something carnivorous in some shape or form. (plant burgers still look like and taste like meat burgers, might as well have the real thing). In fact, transitioning to this kind of diet feels more like getting into something more familiar, more natural.

When you finally decide to get into this kind of diet, the best way to do it is to ease into it slowly but surely. Rather than going cold turkey, start off with your breakfast. If you're not used to eating meat during breakfast, then it is time to create some variations. It would also be best to plan your meals ahead of time and begin to get yourself familiarized with an all-meat breakfast for the next 7 days.

After a week of having an all-meat breakfast, try incorporating all-meat lunches as well. Wait for another week until you are fully immersed into an all-meat food for breakfast and lunch, and then include all-meat dinners. This is only an example. Get creative in your transition, and do whatever works for you.

DISPELLING MYTHS AROUND THE CARNIVORE DIET

1. Eating all-meat can increase your cholesterol levels, leading to cardiac arrest and other heart ailments.

As counterintuitive as it may sound, this diet is highly likely to increase your cholesterol levels, and that is actually a good thing. In truth, there is really no good or bad cholesterol. And it doesn't directly cause heart attacks. Rather, the inflammation of the arterial walls does, and that could be caused by any number of things. In other words, the cholesterol only becomes a big problem when LDL (low density lipoproteins) particles become oxidized or damaged, and then get stuck in your arterial walls.

Also, LDL's play a major role as a part of your body's protection and defense mechanism. They work hand in hand with the immune system to drive out pesky pathogens, and protect you against harmful diseases.

2. Vegetables will complete your nutritional requirement for the day.

Vegetables are good for the body, but that doesn't mean that they are good substitute for animal fats and protein. As mentioned earlier, choline quantities are a big difference between what you get from plant proteins and what you get from animal proteins. Another difference lies in the level of macronutrients provided, which make up your body's daily nutritional requirements.

There are 3 macronutrients, consisting of carbohydrates, protein, and fat. All these are needed for the body to function well. Conversely, there are 4 micronutrients, namely minerals such as Calcium, Potassium, Ionide, Sodium, Magnesium, and Phosphorous. There's vitamins A, B, C, K,

E, Folate, and Choline. There's also amino Acids and Omega 3 and 6 fatty acids.

When you're looking for a healthy diet to adopt, you most likely would be considering factors such as energy supply, nutrient density, as well as any adverse side effects. It is the combination of macro and micro nutrients present, that give you an idea as to the potency of a diet, and when compared side by side, the meat-based meals win every time.

Unfortunately, people have been brainwashed that meat is somewhat unhealthy, especially when matched with kale and broccoli. Biochemically, meats are the only sources where macro and micronutrient are both present.

It is believed that humans can survive by just consuming meats alone. This cannot be said for either carbohydrates or plants. Animal meats have more of the important nutrients except for Vitamin C.

3. The carnivore diet is not safe

This diet is similar to the keto diet mainly because the aim is to eliminate as many carbs from your daily food as possible. And since it has been proven that meat consumption does not directly cause heart ailments, it is fine to say that an all-meat diet is safe.

Also, the idea that the meat you consume will often get stuck in the gastrointestinal tract is not true. Another generalization. Just like with any other food, meat is absorbed and digested in the small intestines, right before it gets in contact with the colon. Though it is possible to experience bowel obstruction, eating red meat does not block the GI tract.

4. Increases inflammation

This is another misconception about the carnivore diet. As proof that this diet will help you fight inflammation, a Boston University study was conducted in obese people with the goal of losing 1 lb. per week. They split participants into two groups.

The first group ate food consisting of 55 percent fat-based calories, 10 percent carbs, and 35 percent protein. Group two consumed 25 percent fat-based calories, 60 percent carbs, and 15 percent protein.

After 12 weeks, scientists measured participants' body composition and weight, and tested blood levels. Group one had a drop of almost 30 percent in their C-reactive protein levels, while the other group only had 3 percent reduction. And so, they came to the conclusion that the fewer carbs you take, the less inflammation you will have, and the better health you will experience.

5.   Meat is not good for the bones

Many people believe that an all meat diet can lead to osteoporosis. According to a theory, when we consume meat, the acid load in the body is increased. The calcium will be moved from the bones and then towards the bloodstream in order to counteract the acid.

While there are short term researches that say meat can cause calcium loss, there are also long-term studies stipulating that meat essentially has significant benefits on bone health.

Bottom line here is regardless of any calcium loss in the short term, a high protein intake helps lower the risk of osteoporosis, and improves bone density in the long term.

GUT BIOMES AND THE CARNIVORE DIET

This diet, much like any other is not without its major criticisms. They range from severe cravings for carbs during the adaptation phase, to stomach upsets, to awkward social situations where the individual is singled out for their carnivorous tastes. One of the most prominent of them however, is its relationship with gut biomes and colon cancer.

It's been said in some studies that those who switched from a high fiber diet to a high protein one, have reportedly observed certain changes to their microbiomes. This is largely influenced by the idea that a diet as restrictive as the carnivore's, only leaves your gut open to the actions of putrefactive bacteria.

The bacteria cause a multiplicity of fermentable fibers, contributing to a more aggressive gut environment and are known to be damaging to the DNA found in your colon cells. And so, it is in light of these discoveries that the probable connection between colon cancer and frequent red meat consumption, has continued to be furthered in discussion.

The following observations have been made with regards to the consumption of animal meat only for 24 hours:
- Significant increase in a bacterium powerfully linked with the development of Crohn's disease, inflammatory bowel diseases, and ulcerative colitis. This bacterium is called Bilophila wadsworthia.
- Significant change in the microbiome.
- Increased resistance to antibiotics in the gut.
- Enhanced development of inflammatory bacteria such as Bilophila, Alistipes, and Bacteroides, and reduced anti-inflammatory bacteria such as Eubacterium rectale, Roseburia, and Ruminococcus bromii.

- Increasing number of secondary bile salts, which are then main causes of liver and colon cancer.
-

To counteract the doomsday talk, it has to be said that as a short-term intervention, removal of the microbiome is always an option, just as long as you replenish the gut with variety of bacteria. Also, it's almost always a case of undigested meat which ferments in the colon and leads to a leaky gut.

Cook your meat properly and that should stave off at least 80 percent of the risk.

THE CARNIVORE DIET AND INTERMITTENT FASTING

The combination of intermittent fasting and carnivore diet has managed to garner a huge following. With people seeing tremendous results in carnivore diet such as fat loss, enhanced mental focus, strength gains, improved allergies, and more energy, it's no wonder that many people are following this all animal diet and fasting combo.

Speaking of intermittent fasting, this unique approach to eating has brought a lot of major health benefits to people such as longevity, disease prevention, fat loss, and confidence. The protocol involved is generally easy, but not for everyone. However, backed by popular opinion, intermittent fasting is said to be a lot easier when paired with the carnivore diet.

Combining the two can be done in 6 ways, they include:

1. **The 5:2 strategy**

This means eating for 5 days on a normal level and then restricting caloric intake to 500 for two days of the week. On your fasting days, women are only allowed to eat 500 calories, while for men, they are only allowed to eat 600 calories.

2.   **The 16/8 Method**

This is done by fasting for 14-16 hours every day, thereby limiting your eating time to only 8-10 hours in a day. Within these eating hours, you can squeeze in at least 2-3 meals. This is considered to be the simplest among all types of intermittent fasting, because you would just skip eating dinner like most would normally do, and then skip breakfast as well. Therefore, your first meal of the day would fall at lunch time.

3.   **Eat-Stop-Eat**

This is also known as a 24-hour fast that can be done once or twice a week. This method lets you fast from breakfast today, till the next breakfast the next day, or from dinner today, up until dinner the next day. Whichever schedule is more suitable for your lifestyle. The end result will still be the same.

Also, during the fast, you are only allowed to drink water and other non-caloric beverages. Solid foods are forbidden.

If you are trying to lose weight and choose this method, make sure to eat the same kind of food that you would normally eat on a typical day during eating periods.

The main challenge most people face with this method of fasting is that a 24-hour fast without eating anything could be a little difficult. But you don't need to go all the way. Assess yourself and see if you can last for 24 hours. If not, you can still go for 14-16 hours of fasting. That still counts.

4. Alternate-Day fasting

This simply means that you will fast every other day. During fasting days, you are only allowed to consume 500 calories. This method may be a bit extreme especially for beginners.

5. Spontaneous Fasting

With this method of intermittent fasting, all you have to do is skip meals periodically or whenever you think will be convenient for you. So, if you're not really hungry, you may choose to skip meals for as long as you can. Just make sure to eat healthy on your next meals.

Chapter 2 – Understanding Meat

In this chapter, I will go full Master Yoda and say that in order to fully understand the carnivore diet, one must first understand the meat itself. This is necessary because understanding and learning the basics and all there is to know about meats, can help improve how you cook and prepare it.

We'll start off with age.

Ageing Beef

This is the process of holding meat for an extended period of time, from the date that they were slaughtered, up until they are prepared on the table and consumed. It may sound unpleasant, but when you say ageing meat, it simply means that it is controlled decomposition. Much like with wine, this is done to improve the taste of the meat, and also enhance its tenderness. It's a process that usually takes 12–14 days.

There are primarily two kinds of ageing meat:

1. Wet ageing

This refers to products that are vacuum-packed and literally "wet" as it sits in its own liquids. This process is considered to be the cheapest and fastest way to age meat. It is also believed to be most cost effective, since there are no losses at all, and you just allow the meat to shrink.
The only setback to this method is the shorter shelf life before the meat deteriorates, further aggravated by any ceaseless closing and opening of the fridge where it is stored. When meat is wet aged for a long period of time, the taste becomes sour and the texture different. The movement from one freezer to another also makes the meat more liquid, and the texture spongier.

2. Dry ageing

This process is done by having the meat exposed to a meticulously controlled environment with levelled humidity and temperature. The tenderness is likewise increased during the process, and the flavor intensified by means of oxidation, a combination of bacteria, and enzyme breakdown.
This process is somewhat expensive due to the use of an equipment, and the final product is often trimmed and shrunk in volume. However, when it reaches the 60-day mark and counting, it undergoes a transformation that is not far removed from that of cheese. The more it ages, the stinkier it gets.
So, what is the best method to take? When you try to differentiate the two, take note that wet ageing only influences the tenderness of the meat, whereas dry ageing affects both tenderness and taste.

Marbling

This is the term used to indicate the quality of a meat. It is an industry term coined to refer to delicate fat lines in meat known as the intramuscular fat. This fat forms within the muscle itself. Intermuscular, on the other hand, is the fat formed between muscles, also known as seam fat.
It is important to take note of marbling because then you will know the quality of the meat you're getting, and that influences the degree of both flavor and tenderness. As a matter of fact, the majority of international meat-grading systems have this as their key element in grade influence, together with other variables.
In general, marbling is important especially when it comes to heritage breeds of pork and beef. This is why Japanese wagyu beef is so expensive, due to its extraordinary genetic predisposition caused by intense marbling.

The Importance of Cutting against the Grain

Another thing to consider in your quest for meat knowledge, is proper slicing. It is always advised to slice it against the grain. However, most people ask how to find the grain and why it is important. Well, that's easy, each muscle of meat contains fibers that run alongside one another in a single direction. That is called the grain.

You can find the grain in meat cuts such as tri-tip, flank, and skirt. However, there are those meat cuts that have several muscles and have different directions of grain such as large cut meats and brisket.

Finding and cutting against the grain means slicing at the right angles where the fibers run. When you cut properly against the grain, it lessens the resistance when eating and chewing the meat, which makes a big difference in its tenderness.

Resting Meat

You can find this instruction in almost all meat recipes stating the importance of resting the meat after cooking. If you have ever seen cooked meat cut, and the juices flowing all over it, that overflow is the exact reason why you need to rest the meat before carving.

Muscles in meat consist of compactly packed protein strands that are squeezed tighter when heated, and its liquids are pressed to the edges when cooking. Resting the meat lets fibers sit and restore moisture to the strands, and evenly redistribute it.

Resting time depends on the kind of recipe you have. A slow cooked roast requires 30 minutes rest, while a quick pan seared steak only takes about 10 minutes.

The Maillard Reaction

This is often identified by a well-browned exterior meat crust, as seen on patties and steaks especially. The act of browning the meat in this manner is known as the Maillard reaction. Every successful sear not only improves the texture and color of the meat, it likewise makes the taste flavorful and makes for an attractive aroma.

The Maillard reaction is a kind of chemical reaction between sugars and amino acids. This is different from ordinary browning and usually difficult to achieve, but the one factor that makes all the difference is moisture. In Maillard, you eliminate as much moistness as possible before cooking.

This reaction often takes place in high heat and dry conditions. So before searing, it is advised to completely dry and pat the meat with paper towels, to make sure that everything else is dry.

ALL ABOUT MEAT TEMPERATURE

No matter which method of cooking you choose, whether slow and low, the most significant factor to consider when cooking meat is the temperature. For instance, it's commonly accepted that pork shoulders need to reach at least 88°C or 190°F before it becomes tender and readily edible. Below are some of the variables which you might want to consider, the next time you are cooking meat.

Grill temperatures

Grill means direct heat gas unit or coal. If you don't have a temperature gauge available, you can use the hand method. This gauges how many seconds you can hold your hand over the heat before you need to draw your hand out.

Accuracy

When it comes to cooking meat, there are just about as many kinds of variables to consider. Are you cooking grain? How thick is the cut? Which cooking method to use? How about the heat source? the temperature? Despite the many influencing factors, cooking to temperature is always reliable. This is also important in maintaining food safety, as pork and chicken need to achieve a certain kind of internal temperature to kill bacteria, and make sure they are safe for consumption.

Doneness

This is the degree by which the meat is cooked. Doneness is mostly associated with steaks (rare, medium, or well done) although these can all be associated in almost all kinds of meat. You may need to invest in a meat thermometer to gauge doneness.

Speaking of doneness, you might be asking, how about the "rare" burger? It would be horrifying to look at a patty that's pink in the middle. This is the reason why people eat rare steaks.

Here's a doneness chart to serve as guide:
Rare - 125–130°F of 52–54°C
Medium Rare - 130–135°F or 54–57°C
Medium - 135–145°F or 57–63°C
Medium well - 145–155°F or 63–68°C
Well done - 155°F+ or 68°C+

Chapter 3 – Different Ways to Cut Meat

You definitely don't need the chopping skills of Nusret Gokce aka *Salt Bae* on your carnivore diet journey, but there are basic techniques which you can learn and employ to add a little finesse to your meat cutting, and with constant practice, you too can be slicing meat into as many cuts as you desire, as a neat party trick.

Some of them include:

The Butterfly Cut and Truss a Loin

This is considered to be the most basic way of cutting meat. In fact, from the moment you learn how to butterfly a loin, it automatically becomes easier to cut large chunks of meat.

Butterflying has 3 major cuts that are similar to a narrow U shape. To execute any one of them, you would need a butcher's twine, a boning knife and the following instructions:

1. To make the first cut, from the bottom of the loin, cut about ½ inch, stopping first before you make a cut all the way through.
2. To make the cut ship-shaped, cut in one motion only instead of making too many small cuts. This will give your butterfly cut a more professional look.
3. Follow the curve of the loin as you continue to make the cut.
4. For the final cut, you will open up the piece of the meat into one even slab.
5. If you are to put some stuffing, you can arrange them across the length of the meat.
6. Measure before cutting a part of the twine 2-3 times the length of the meat.

7. Cutting from left to the right, cut at least ¾ inches from the edge, and then secure with a loop.
8. Loop the twine around the meat once again, then pass the twine's end from left to right beneath the loop. To secure, pull the loop.
9. Continue with the process as you make some even spacing on the loops.
10. When the end of the meat is reached, tie the last loop on the right side. You also have the option of tying the loop one at a time instead of doing them in one single piece.

Flattening a Chicken

This is also called as spatchcocking or the flattening of meat to make cooking more even. It is done using the following steps:
1. You will need paper towels and kitchen shears.
2. First, you need to eliminate the giblets and other stuff inside the chicken cavity.
3. Put the chicken breast side down on a board. Cut up one side of the backbone using kitchen shears.
4. Slice along the other side and then remove the backbone.
5. Flip the chicken over and break the breastbone. Tuck the wings to flatten the chicken.
6. Your chicken is now spatchcocked and ready to cook.

Grinding Your Own Meat Burger

If you are going to make the carnivore diet a lifetime diet, grinding meat for your burgers will come in handy if you know how to. It's also important so you have full control of the quality as well as the flavor. Some of the meats to grind are short rib, round, brisket, and chuck. Premium cuts such as rib eye and tenderloin are a no-no.

It is also important to note that the texture and fat ratio of the meat will have more to do with the taste than the cut itself. So, no matter which cut you opt for, ensure that the final grind contains at least 20 percent fat to yield a juicy outcome.

When you grind the meat, make sure that both the meat and the grinder are cold. If both heat up too much, the meat's texture will be affected. Take note of the following steps:

1. To cool the grinder before using, place it in the freezer for at least an hour.
2. Cut the meat off any connective tissue, and then cube it. The size must be at least 2-3 centimeters. Return to the fridge and allow to cool for at least 1 hour before grinding.
3. After an hour, pass the meat through the grinder and then mince. Work as quickly as possible to retain the cold temperature.
4. Return newly minced meat back to the fridge for 1 hour before forming them into patties. Do not put salt just yet. Wait until you are in the cooking process before you season the patties.

Chapter 4 – Seasoning Meat

Both temperature and the presence of salt as seasoning exert major influence on how meat will taste. Seasoning meat makes all the difference between flavorsome and bland, and we are going to start of with the most basic of seasonings for meat, which is salt.

Salt

Table salt is essentially an antimicrobial compound also known as sodium chloride, and can be used as a preservative in addition to its seasoning function. The moment you sprinkle some of it onto the meat, liquid is drawn out via the process of osmosis and towards the salt's crystals. It produces a slimy and watery surface that ultimately liquefies the salt crystals, and if set aside for a long period of time, draws the salty brine back into the meat via diffusion.

It is important to note that all salts are not equal, and some are made brinier than their counterparts. This just means that it's rare for any two types or brands of salt to have the same degree of potency.
Despite all salts having a similar compound, the disparity arises from its density, or the amount of air or space contained in each crystal. This dictates the amount of sodium chloride that actually comprises that crystal. And so, the bigger the quantity per crystal, the higher the potency.

Salt also plays a role as a tenderizer and destroy the proteins' characteristic properties in order to effectively loosen the strings from one another. This makes for a more tender meat.

Deep seasoning

Dry brining or deep seasoning is the popular way to season your meat with salt. With dry brining, all you do is sprinkle salt onto the meat and leave it for a few hours, uncovered on a rack above in a drip tray. Place inside the fridge until ready to cook.

The concept here is to let the salty brine be absorbed by the meat completely, and at the same time have a drying effect on the outside. This method helps in making a crusty texture on the outside, but tender on the inside.

When you deep season, it has a good effect on both tenderness and taste of the meat. The following methods will help you get started:
1. Season steak and set aside for at least 24 hours. You can also deep season it for up to 72 hours.
2. The steak should be cut 1 inch thick.
3. Do not put some more salt after deep seasoning.
4. When you deep season, make sure that there is also a baking soda inside the fridge to absorb any odors that may contaminate the meat.

Timing Your Seasoning

The process of denaturing and osmosis take time, so timing is really of the essence. When seasoning, you have 2 options:
1. Salt the meat immediately before cooking AND before the salt has a chance to draw the moisture to the surface and delay the onset of the Maillard reaction.
2. Apply seasoning and leave the meat for about 45 minutes, so any moisture that is drawn to the surface has the opportunity to reabsorb.

Essentially, try to steer clear of salting your meat anywhere during the 10–30 minute mark, prior to cooking. All you'll be doing is drawing moisture out without giving it the opportunity to soak back in.

Chapter 5 – Different Methods of Cooking Meat

The Reverse Sear Method

Without overstating it, the reverse sear method has wholly transformed the way most people cook their steaks nowadays. This method is nearly a proven way to cook medium-rare steak, especially where the pinkness has stayed in perfection from edge to edge without any traces of grey.
By tradition, restaurants would solder steak over an extremely hot surface. They would then place the meat inside the oven to complete the cooking process until the desired temperature was reached. In this method, the meat searing is done in the reverse. The good thing about this is that after the steak is seared, you can already start eating your steak because it has already been rested.
The reverse sear method can be executed regardless of the cut, as long as it is 2.5 centimeters thick. It can also be done in a number of ways which include

Grilling

If you're going to use this method of cooking meat, make sure to arrange your grill to two-zone cooking. Pat the steak dry and season with salt. Place steak indirectly on the grill. Cook until your desired doneness is reached. Remove from the grill and let the meat rest for 15 minutes before carving and serving.

Pan and Oven

Preheat the oven to 275°F or 135°C. Make sure to pat the steak dry and season with salt. Place the steak on a baking pan and place inside the oven. Cook until the meat reaches your

preferred internal temperature. This will take between 45 minutes to 1 hour. Let steak rest for 15 minutes.
If you're going to use a pan, place a heavy-based pan set over high heat. Let the pan reach its smoking point. Sear the steak for 2 minutes per side. Serve in an instant.

Smoker

Heat a smoker to 275°F or 135°C. Make sure to pat the steak dry and season with salt. Place the steak in the smoker. Cook until your preferred internal temperature is achieved. Let meat rest for 15 minutes and then serve.
The steak requires that it be seared over high temperature. This can be on a pan, hot grill, or stove. Sear for 2 minutes per side, and then serve.

Different Types of Smokers

Electric smoker

Electric smokers come with a box for wood shavings and heating element. This kind of smoker is short of combustion, and so meats cooked on an electric smoker lack flavor. The smolders leave the meat with a pungent taste. Yes, the smoker may have produced a smoked meat, but nothing compares to the conventional barbecue.

Pellet grill

This type of smoker has a built-in thermostat that lets you set the exact temperature. The grill is powered by compact wood pellets that ignite to produce smoke, are pushed by an auger, and held in a hopper. The smoke can be very mild, so much so that you would occasionally need a smoker tube to increase the smokiness of the cooked meat. This grill runs on electricity so you would probably need an extension cord for this. Also, be prepared for possible repairs that may be a bit pricey and complicated. As for the food that this type of smoker produces, some units find it hard to get it enough hot to properly sear meat.

Charcoal grill

This kind of grill can be transformed into a decent smoker. All you have to do is have the coals stacked around the edge of the grill and make sure that only one end is ignited.
A charcoal smoker may take a long time to cook meat, as this resembles barbecuing at low heat. The downside of this is that you would have to continuously refill the charcoal to ensure that it would last until your cooking is done. It also has limited space, so you will find it a bit challenging to set aside some meat that only needs heating in a few specific areas.

The offset pit

This is considered to be the most commonly used, but is a bit hard to master. However, this kind of grill generates excellent results when used the right way. It is fired up wholly by using wood logs and the heat is controlled manually. Unlike the other units of smokers that only require very little amount of wood for extra flavor, the offset pit produces both smoke and heat from logs for added flavor.
However, you must take note that this type of smoker requires hard work to run and may also take some getting used to, especially in terms of controlling the temperature sans the spikes. Given the amount of effort that goes into operating this smoker, the saving solace is that it yields flavorful meats with natural rings and bark, or the exterior crust.

Bullet smoker

As the name implies, this smoker is shaped like a bullet, making it easier to place, especially in a limited space. The water found at the base will help keep the moisture the entire time, thereby preventing your meat from lacking fluids.

Much like other grills, the heat comes from the charcoal. If you want to produce smoke, you will be needing more wood chips and chunks to be placed on the coals.

Chapter 5 – Carnivore Recipes

1. Southern Deviled Eggs

Ingredients:
- 4 hard-boiled eggs, peeled
- 1/4 cup of mayonnaise
- Salt
- pepper to taste
- Paprika, for garnish

Directions:
1. Halve the eggs lengthwise and then remove yolks and transfer to a small bowl.
2. Use a fork to mash egg yolks and mayonnaise. Season with salt and pepper.
3. Spoon in the yolk mixture into the egg whites, making sure it is divided evenly.
4. Use paprika to garnish. Keep covered in the fridge.

2. Unsweetened Mustard Baked Ham

Ingredients:
- 15 pounds whole bone-in ham
- ½ cup unsweetened mustard, carnivore-friendly
- 4 cups brown erythritol

Directions:
1. In a mixing bowl, combine mustard and erythritol until it becomes a thick paste.
2. Trim away excess fat off the ham.
3. Line baking pan with aluminum foil.
4. Place ham on foil and spread the mustard/ erythritol paste on top.
5. Fold and seal foil. Bake at 350 degrees Fahrenheit for 4 hours.
6. Rest for 1 hour and carve.

3. Breakfast Sausage and Cheese Casserole

Ingredients:
- 6 large eggs
- 1 pound breakfast sausage
- 1 container cottage cheese
- 12 ounces mild Cheddar cheese
- 1/2 cup onion
- 1/4 cup butter

Directions:
1. Preheat your oven to 375 degrees F.
2. Prepare a square baking dish and grease it olive or vegetable oil.
3. Cook the breakfast sausage in olive oil until golden brown, crumble into small pieces and set aside.
4. Use a grater to shred the potatoes, add butter and set aside in a small bowl.
5. In a mixing bowl, combine the crumbled breakfast sausages, onion, cheddar cheese, cottage cheese and 6 beaten large eggs.
6. Use the potato mixture and fold it with the sausages, and then transfer all into a baking dish.
7. Bake the sausage batter in the oven for 1 hour then allot an extra 5 minutes for it to cool.
8. Serve the 2-Cheese Breakfast Sausage Casserole with garlic bread sticks and enjoy.

4. Sausage Burger Patty

Ingredients:
- 1 pinch cloves
- 2 pounds ground pork
- 1 tablespoon erythritol
- 2 teaspoons sage
- 1/4 teaspoon marjoram
- 1/8 teaspoon red pepper flakes
- 2 teaspoons salt

- 1 teaspoon black pepper

Directions:
1. In a small bowl, mix salt, marjoram, ground black pepper, sage, crushed red pepper, cloves, and erythritol.
2. In a large bowl, mix the pork and all the dried spices and shape them into burger patties.
3. In a skillet, sauté the pork patties and cook for 5 minutes.
4. Once the patties are cooked, serve on a plate with bread and chips.

5. Roasted Pork Tacos

Ingredients:
- 1 ½ tsp salt to taste
- 1 tsp taco seasoning
- ¼ cup chilli powder
- 4 pork shoulder roast
- 2 tsp garlic, minced
- 1 tsp dried oregano
- 2 4 oz cans diced green chillies, drained

Directions:
1. Set the oven at 300 degrees.
2. Place the roast on top of an aluminum foil. Combine the green chillies, oregano, garlic, chilli powder and taco seasoning.
3. Rub the mixture over the roast. Wrap the foil around the roast tightly to make sure that it is completely covered. You can use additionally foil if necessary.
4. Place it in a roasting rack. Place a baking sheet underneath to catch any dripping.
5. Roast for 3 1/2 – 4 hours until the meat is falling apart. Cook at 145 degrees. Transfer it to a plate and shred to smaller pieces using knife or fork. Add salt and toss to season.

6. Steak Tacos

Ingredients:
- 2 lb top sirloin steak, cut into thin strips
- 18 tortillas
- Salt
- Pepper to taste
- 1 onion, diced
- ¼ cup cooking oil
- 4 limes cut into wedges

Directions:
1. Place a large pan on top of medium heat. Add the steak and cook until it is browned on the outside. This should take about 5 minutes.
2. Season the steak with salt and pepper. Place it in a plate and cover to keep the dish warm.
3. Add oil to the same pan. Heat it for a few minutes. Place the tortilla in the pan and cook. Flip it once and cook until the tortilla is slightly browned.
4. Repeat the same process for the remaining tortillas.
5. Place the tortilla in a serving plate. To serve, squeeze limes and spread the juice on top of the steak. Serve it warm.

7. Baked Chicken and Eggs

Ingredients:
- ½ tbsp. olive oil
- 2 garlic cloves, chopped
- 1 can tomato juices
- Handful of basil leaves, shredded
- 2 eggs
- ¼ cup chicken strips

Directions:
1. Preheat the oven to 350 degrees F.

2.   Pour olive oil into the skillet. Once hot, saute garlic and pour tomato juices.
3.   Secure the lid and allow mixture to simmer for 10 minutes.
4.   Meanwhile, place chicken strips in a baking dish. Crack the eggs. Season with salt and pepper.
5.   Place baking dish inside the microwave oven. Heat for 10 minutes. Serve.

8. Tuna Omelet

Ingredients:
- 3 eggs, whisked
- 1 can canned tuna flakes in oil, drained
- Pinch of garlic salt
- 1 Tbsp. olive oil
- Pinch of black pepper, to taste

Directions:
1.   Put together eggs, tuna flakes, garlic salt, and pepper into a bowl. Set aside.
2.   Meanwhile, pour olive oil into the skillet. Once hot, pour the omelet mixture. Swirl the skillet to evenly distribute the ingredients.
3.   Cook the eggs until the middle is no longer wobbly and the edges are set.
4.   Remove from the skillet. Slice and serve.

9. Egg Cups

Ingredients:
- 3 eggs
- 6 streaky bacon strips
- Pinch of sea salt
- Pinch of black pepper, to taste
- Dried chili flakes, optional

Directions:
1. Preheat the oven to 400°F. Put 3 laminated paper liners into 3 muffin tins. Put green beans into the paper liners.
2. Layer 2 bacon strips on the side of the paper liner. Make sure to overhang bacon so that they won't fold during the baking process.
3. Crack an egg into the muffin tin. Season with salt and pepper. Bake for 12 minutes or until the bacon is crisp and the eggs are set.
4. Remove muffin tin from the oven. Serve egg cups in paper liners.

10. Turkey Omelet

Ingredients:
- 3 oz of lean ground turkey
- 1 whole egg
- 4 egg whites
- 1 oz of goat cheese
- 1 oz of goat cheese

Directions:
1. Season the ground turkey with salt and pepper. Set aside.
2. Pour olive oil in a pan over medium heat. Cook the egg whites and whole egg.
3. Stir in ground turkey and cheese. Mix well.
4. Place mixture in a plastic wrap. Slice into four.
5. Put inside the fridge for 24 hours, or until ready to cook. You can make this ahead of time. Serve as needed.

11. Scotch Eggs and Sausage

Ingredients:
- 6 eggs, hardboiled
- 1 ½ tsp. garlic powder

- 1 ½ cups sausage
- 1/3 tsp. sea salt
- ½ tsp. ground black pepper

Directions:
1. Preheat the oven to 400 degrees F to preheat. Spread a large sheet of baking paper on a dry surface.
2. Meanwhile, put sausage in a bowl. Season with garlic powder, salt, and pepper. Mix using your hands.
3. Divide breakfast sausage mixture into equal balls. Arrange on the baking sheet. Flatten sausage balls. Put hardboiled egg on top. Wrap the egg with sausage mixture.
4. Layer sausage-coated eggs on a baking sheet. Place inside the oven and bake for 25 minutes.
5. Let cool for 5 minutes. Store in an airtight container. This will keep for 4 days.

12. Ham and Egg Cups

Ingredients:
- 1 thick sugar-free sourdough bread, quartered
- 4 slices sweet ham, sliced into slivers
- 10 quail eggs
- 2 tsp. cheddar cheese, grated
- Pinch of white pepper, to taste

Directions:
1. Preheat the oven to 350°F. Place 5 paper liners into muffin tins. Set aside.
2. Put bread quarter into the base of each muffin cup. Break 2 quail eggs and sweet ham on top of the bread.
3. Scatter grated cheddar cheese. Bake for 15 minutes or until set. Remove muffin tins from the oven and allow to cool at room temperature.
4. Remove cup from tins. Season with pepper. Serve.

LUNCH RECIPES

13. Crispy Chicken and Pork Rind in Lettuce Wraps

Ingredients:
Dipping sauce
- 1 garlic clove, minced
- ¼ tsp ginger, grated
- 1 red chili, minced
- ½ cup apple cider vinegar
- 1 Tbsp. oyster sauce
- 3 Tbsp. soy sauce
- 1 Tbsp. honey

Crispy chicken
- olive oil
- 2 chicken thigh fillets, sliced lengthwise
- Pinch of sea salt, add more if needed
- Dash of Spanish paprika
- ½ tsp. almond flour

- 4 pork rind cracklings, lightly crushed

Directions:
1. For the chicken, pour olive oil into the skillet. Season chicken thigh fillets with salt and Spanish paprika.
2. For the dipping sauce, put together garlic, ginger, chili, apple cider vinegar, oyster sauce, soy sauce, and honey in a bowl.
3. Dredge chicken fillets into almond flour. Fry until fillets are golden brown on all sides. Damp in paper towels to remove excess grease.
4. To assemble, place fried chicken and dipping sauce into individual plates. Add a piece of crackling. Serve with dipping sauce.

14 - Chicken with Yogurt Sauce

Ingredients:
- 3 chicken breasts, boneless, skinless
- 1 cup chicken stock, divided
- 2 garlic cloves, minced
- 2 ½ Tbsp. plain Greek yogurt, low-fat
- Pinch of sea salt
- Pinch of ground black pepper, to taste

Directions:
1. Season chicken breast with salt and pepper.
2. Pour chicken broth in a large saucepan. Add in chicken breast. Allow to simmer for 10 minutes.
3. Stir in garlic. Pour the remaining chicken stock. Cover and cook for another 5 minutes.
4. Meanwhile, put yogurt in a bowl. Mix well.
5. Once the chicken broth has dried out, pour the yogurt mixture into the saucepan. Mix. Reduce the heat and allow to simmer for 5 minutes. Serve.

15. Curried Salmon

Ingredients:
- 3 salmon fillets, skinless
- ¾ cup chicken stock, low-sodium
- 1 ½ cups evaporated milk
- 1 Tbsp. red curry paste
- 1 garlic clove, minced
- 1 fresh ginger, minced
- 1 red chili pepper, thinly sliced
- ¾ Tbsp. organic fish sauce
-

Directions:
1. Mix the chicken stock, evaporated milk, and curry paste into the saucepan. Add in salmon fillets.

2.   Stir in garlic, ginger, and chili pepper. Season with fish sauce. Mix until all ingredients are well incorporated.
3.   Cover and cook for 30 minutes. Reduce the heat and allow to simmer for 20 minutes or until the sauce thickens. Serve.

16. Beef Stew

Ingredients:
- ¾ lb beef stew, chopped into 2-inch cubes, create slits all over
- 2 Tbsp. olive oil
- 1 yellow onion, thinly sliced
- 8 garlic cloves, slivered
- 1/3 cup dry red wine vinegar
- 1 cinnamon stick
- ¾ tsp smoked paprika
- ½ cup Pecorino Romano cheese, grated
- 1 tsp sea salt
- ½ tsp freshly ground black pepper

Directions:
1.   Stuff beef cubes with slivered garlic. Season with salt and pepper.
2.   Place a stock pot over medium flame and heat the oil. Brown the beef all over, then place on a platter.
3.   Sauté the onion in the stockpot until golden brown. Add the vinegar, then return the beef. Increase to high flame and sauté until vinegar evaporates.
4.   Stir in cinnamon stick and paprika. Sauté to combine.
5.   Cover the pot and reduce to medium low flame. Simmer for about 1 hour 30 minutes, adding ½ cup water every 15 to 20 minutes, or until meat is extra tender.
6.   To serve, ladle the sauce over the cooked pasta, then top with cheese.

17. Chicken Curry

Ingredients:
- ½ lb. chicken breast, sliced into thin strips
- ¼ cup yellow onion, diced
- 1 garlic clove, minced
- 1 tsp. fresh ginger, minced
- 7.5 oz. evaporated milk, full fat, unsweetened
- ½ Tbsp. curry powder
- ¼ cup water
- 3 Tbsp. cooking oil
- Pinch of sea salt, to taste
- Dash of red pepper flakes

Directions:
1. Pour cooking oil in a saucepan set over medium heat.
2. Saute onion, garlic, and ginger for 2 minutes or until limp and fragrant. Add in curry powder.
3. Stir in chicken. Cook until tender. Pour evaporated milk and water. Bring mixture to a boil.
4. Once boiling, reduce the heat and allow to simmer. Continue cooking until the sauce is thickened and the chicken cooked through.
5. Remove from heat. Season with salt and red pepper flakes. Serve.
6. For leftovers, store in airtight containers. Let cool before placing inside the fridge. This will keep for 3 days. Reheat before serving.

18. Slow Cooked Creamy Sausage

Ingredients:
- 1 cup broccoli chopped
- 1 cup sausage, sliced, cooked
- 1 cup cheddar cheese, shredded
- Pinch of salt
- ½ tbsp. pepper
- 2 garlic cloves, minced

- 1 cup whipping cream
- 8 eggs

Directions:
1. Arrange half of the sausage and cheese in the slow cooker. Top with another layer of the rest of the sausage, and cheese.
2. Meanwhile, combine whipping cream, garlic, eggs, salt, and pepper in a bowl. Place mixture in the slow cooker.
3. Cover and cook for 2 hours and 30 minutes, undisturbed. Serve.

19. Rosemary and Thyme Pork Tenderloin

Ingredients:
- ¾ lb. pork tenderloin, sliced into thick medallions
- 3 fresh thyme sprigs
- 3 fresh rosemary sprigs
- 1 ½ Tbsp. olive oil
- 1 garlic clove, minced
- 1 shallot, minced
- 3 Tbsp. butter
- 2 Tbsp. balsamic vinegar
- ¾ tsp. soy sauce
- Pinch of sea salt, to taste
- Pinch of ground black pepper, to taste

Directions:
1. Preheat the oven to 475 degrees F. Season pork medallions with salt and pepper.
2. Pour olive oil in an ovenproof skillet set over medium heat. Once hot, saute shallot and garlic until fragrant. Add pork medallions. Sear for 2 minutes on each side.
3. Stir in soy sauce, balsamic vinegar, remaining butter thyme, and rosemary. Mix well. Spoon mixture over the pork. Cook for 2 minutes.

4.   Place inside the oven and bake for 5 minutes. Turn over pork medallions and cook for an additional 5 minutes.
5.   Transfer to a platter. Let rest for 3 minutes. Spoon sauce on top.
6.   For leftovers, this can keep in the fridge for 3 days.

20. Spicy Shrimps

Ingredients:
- 20 pcs raw shrimp, deveined
- 4 garlic cloves, minced
- 1 onion, halved, thinly sliced
- 2 jalapeno peppers, thinly sliced
- 1 lime, cut into wedges
- 2 tsp olive oil

Directions:
1.   Heat olive oil in a big non-stick skillet over medium fire. Put in the bay leaf and cook for one minute.
2.   Sauté the jalapeno, onion and garlic for around 3 minutes. Stir constantly until the ingredients have become softened.
3.   Stir in the shrimps. Cover the skillet and cook for three to four minutes or until the shrimps are pink or thoroughly cooked.
4.   Stir in the olives and tomatoes.
5.   Allow the mixture to simmer and lower the heat to medium. Put back the cover. Discard bay leaf.
6.   Serve with lime wedges.

21. Ginger Meatballs

Ingredients:
- ☐   1½ pounds lean ground pork
- ☐   2 eggs, whisked, use only 1 yolk
- ☐   3 Tbsp. fresh ginger, grated
- ☐   3 Tbsp. fresh coriander, minced

- ☐ Pinch of sea salt
- ☐ Pinch of black pepper, to taste

Directions:
1. Fill the steamer with water of about ¾ full. Close the lid. Bring water to a rolling boil.
2. Meanwhile, grease the sides and bottom of a steaming basket with coconut oil.
3. Put together lean ground pork, eggs, ginger, coriander, salt, and pepper in a mixing bowl.
4. Roll into balls and place in the steaming basket. Steam meatballs for 45 minutes.
5. Turn off the heat. Layer meatballs in a platter.

22. Burrito Steak

Ingredients:
- 12 oz. strip steak, cut into thin slices
- ½ cup fresh salsa
- ½ cup water
- ¼ tsp ground pepper
- 4 tortilla
- 1 tbsp. olive oil
- ¼ cup prepared guacamole
- ½ cup cheddar cheese, shredded

Directions:
1. Mix water and salsa in a small saucepan and allow to boil.
2. Stir in the brown rice. Lower the heat to let the mixture simmer. Cover and cook for five minutes.
3. In the meantime, sprinkle the pepper onto the steak.
4. On a large skillet, heat the oil over medium to high fire.
5. Cook the steak for 3 to 5 minutes or until it becomes brown and thoroughly cooked.

6. Assemble the burritos by dividing the steak amongst the four tortillas. Top the steak with equivalent amounts of guacamole, and cheese.
7. Roll the tortillas and wrap in aluminum foil.

23. Spiced Pork and Beef with Cheese

Ingredients:
- 1 ground beef, lean
- 1 ground pork, lean
- 2 Tbsp. olive oil
- ½ streaky bacon, diced
- 1 onion, minced
- 2 garlic cloves, minced
- 1 cup beef broth
- 2 Tbsp. chili powder
- 2 jalapeño pepper, minced
- 1 Tbsp. cayenne powder
- ⅛ Tbsp. black pepper
- Dash of red pepper flakes
- Pinch of sea salt, add more if needed
- 1 package cheddar cheese curds

Directions:
1. Pour olive oil into the saucepan. Cook bacon until crisp. Saute onion and garlic for 2 minutes or until fragrant and translucent.
2. Cook ground beef and pork. Cook until larger clumps are broken and browned all over.
3. Add in beef broth, chili powder, jalapeño pepper, cayenne powder, black pepper, and red pepper flakes. Bring mixture to a rolling boil.
4. Reduce the heat. Allow to simmer for 30 minutes or until the liquid has been reduced. Season with salt. Tip in cheese curds. Serve.

24. Chicken Meatball Soup

Ingredients:
For the Chicken Meatballs
- 1½ pounds lean ground chicken
- ½ tsp. almond flour, finely milled
- 1 egg, whisked, discard yolks
- Pinch of sea salt
- Pinch of black pepper, to taste

- 2 tsp. olive oil
- 2 garlic cloves, minced
- 1 thumb-sized ginger, julienned
- 4 cups chicken broth

Directions:
1. Put together ground chicken, almond flour, egg, chives, salt, and pepper in a mixing bowl. Roll into bite-sized meatballs. Transfer meatballs to the baking sheet. Place in the freezer until ready to cook.
2. Meanwhile, pour olive oil into a large saucepan. Once the oil is hot, saute garlic and ginger for 3 minutes or until the carrots are fork tender.
3. Pour chicken broth. Drop meatballs and allow the mixture to boil. Cook until the chicken meatballs have floated.
4. Remove from heat. Adjust taste if needed. Serve.

25. Chicken in Egg Soup

Ingredients:
- 4 cups chicken broth
- 1 pound chicken thigh fillets, diced
- 2 eggs, whisked, discard yolks
- 2 Tbsp. olive oil
- 2 garlic cloves, grated
- ½ tsp. ginger, grated
- 2 drops olive oil

- ½ tsp. fish sauce
- ½ tsp. Spanish paprika
- Dash of red pepper flakes
- Pinch of sea salt
- Pinch of black pepper, to taste

Directions:
1. Pour olive oil into a Dutch oven. Sauté ginger and garlic for 2 minutes. Pour chicken broth and chicken thigh fillets. Bring mixture to a rolling boil.
2. Reduce the heat and allow to simmer for 20 minutes or until the fillets are fork tender. Season soup with sesame oil, fish sauce, Spanish paprika, red pepper flakes, salt, and pepper. Adjust taste if needed.
3. Turn off the heat. Pour whisked eggs. Stir mixture well. Cook for another 3 minutes with lid on. Allow residual heat to cook the eggs.
4. To serve, ladle an equal amount of soup into bowls.

26. Stuffed Flank Steak

Ingredients:
- ¾ lbs. flank steak, tenderized
- 1 egg, beaten
- 2 tsp. olive oil
- ¼ cup red peppers, jarred, roasted
- ½ yellow onion, thinly sliced
- 1 garlic clove, minced
- ½ cup white wine vinegar
- 1 Tbsp. Parmesan cheese, grated
- ¼ cup feta cheese, crumbled
- ½ tsp. dried basil
- Pinch of sea salt
- Pinch of ground black pepper, to taste

Directions:
1. Preheat the broiler.

2. Add in breadcrumbs in a bowl. Drizzle in olive oil. Toss well.
3. Pour beaten egg and roasted red peppers. Mix well until all ingredients are well combined. Add in Parmesan and feta cheeses.
4. Spread mixture on top of the butterflied flank steak. Season with salt and pepper.
5. Roll up flank steak to make a log. Secure the ends with butcher string.
6. Pour olive oil into the skillet. Once hot, add in rolled steak. Cook for 5 minutes until the meat turns brown.
7. Saute onion, garlic and white wine vinegar.
8. Put steak to a baking dish. Place inside the broiler. Broil for 20 minutes.
9. Transfer steak to a carving board. Let it sit for 5 minutes before slicing. Remove the butcher twine and then slice.
10. Put an equal amount of flank steak into plates. Serve.

27. Beef Balls with Dip

Ingredients:
- 1 lb. ground beef
- 1 red onion, minced
- 2 garlic cloves, minced
- 1 egg
- ½ tsp. sea salt
- Pinch of ground black pepper, to taste

For the Sauce
- 1 garlic clove, minced
- 2 Tbsp. red wine vinegar
- ¼ cup light soy sauce
- 1 Tbsp. ginger, grated
- Liquid stevia
- Nonstick cooking spray

Directions:
1. Preheat the oven to 425 degrees F. Lightly grease a baking sheet with cooking spray. Set aside.
2. Put ground beef in a mixing bowl. Add in onion, garlic, egg, salt, and black pepper. Mix well using your hands.
3. Form mixture into balls. Arrange on the baking sheet.
4. Bake inside the oven for 12 minutes, or until browned all over.
5. Meanwhile, put together all sauce ingredients in a small bowl. Mix well.
6. Transfer meatballs to an airtight container. Let cool before storing in an airtight container. Store the dipping sauce in a separate container.
7. Refrigerate meatballs and sauce for up to 3 days. Reheat before serving.

28. Chicken with Garlic Tomatillo Sauce

Ingredients:

For the Chicken

- 1 lb. chicken breasts
- 1 garlic clove, chopped
- 1/4 yellow onion, finely chopped
- 2 tbsp. olive oil
- Pinch of sea salt

For the Sauce

- 3 garlic cloves, chopped
- 1 Serrano chili
- ½ cup tomatillo sauce
- Pinch of sea salt
- 1/8 cup cooking fat

Directions:

1. Place 2 tablespoons olive oil in a deep frying pan and sauté garlic and onions. Sauté until brown. Season chicken breasts with salt and. Place on heated oil and fry. Cook until both sides are brown in color. Set aside.
2. Put chiles in a saucepan. Pour water until the first ingredients are completely covered by water. Set stove in medium-high heat and bring to a boil. Continue boiling for 15 minutes.
3. Add chilies and garlic to the processor. Process until it forms a smooth, saucy texture.
4. Heat oil in a saucepan. Once it's smoking, add tomatillo sauce. Stir constantly until it simmers and forms small bubbles. Decrease heat and continue simmering for five minutes until the sauce thickens. Add a tablespoon of salt.
5. Drop pre-cooked chicken into the sauce. Continue simmering for 45 minutes until it completely cooks. Scoop out chicken and shred. Measure a cup of sauce for later use.
6. Bring the chicken back and season according to preference. Continue simmering while assembling the meal.

29. Chicken-Ginger Stew

Ingredients:
- Dash of garlic powder
- Dash of onion powder
- ¼ cup chicken thigh fillet, diced
- 1 ginger, crushed
- 1 cup chicken stock
- 1 cup water
- 1 tsp. fish sauce
- 1 bird's eye chili, minced
- Pinch of white pepper

Directions:

1. Put together chicken thigh fillet, ginger, chicken stock, water fish sauce, bird's eye chili, garlic powder, onion powder, and white pepper in a saucepan. Bring to a boil.
2. Once boiling, reduce the heat. Allow stew to simmer for 20 minutes or until the papaya is tender and the chicken fillet is cooked through. Serve hot.

30. Turkey Chicken Chorizo

Ingredients:
- 2½ pounds lean chicken thighs
- 4 links turkey chorizos, links separated
- 1 garlic bulb, cloves separated
- 1 tsp. unsweetened mustard
- 1 lemon, freshly squeezed ¼ cup olive oil
- Pinch of sea salt
- Pinch of black pepper to taste

Directions:
1. Preheat the oven to 425°F. Line a roasting tin with aluminum foil.
2. Put garlic bulb, mustard, lean chicken thighs, olive oil, salt, and pepper in freezer-safe bag. Seal the bag and marinate the chicken for 2 hours or until ready to use.
3. Pour contents of the bag into the prepared roasting tin. Arrange chicken thighs on the baking surface skin side up. Tuck turkey chorizos in between the chicken. Place another layer of aluminum foil. Bake for 1 hour.
4. Remove the foil. Bake the chicken for another 15 minutes. Remove from the oven. Let cool for a few minutes before serving.

31. Spicy Clams and Bacon

Ingredients:
- 2 dozen clams, shucked
- 4 slices bacon, finally chopped

- 2 tablespoons olive oil
- 1 garlic clove, minced
- 1 onion, minced
- ¼ teaspoon salt
- ¼ teaspoon pepper

Directions:
1. Preheat the grill to medium-high.
2. Meanwhile, in a nonstick skillet, heat the oil over medium heat. Add the garlic, onion, bacon, salt, and pepper. Cook for 7 minutes or until the bacon is tender and other vegetables softened.
3. Remove from the skillet and stir parsley and lemon zest.
4. Place each clam and pour the bacon mixture. Grill clams and cover until cooked through. Serve.

32. Garlicy Turkey Chunks

Ingredients:

- 2 lbs turkey chunks, thinly sliced
- 2 tablespoons olive oil
- 2 cloves garlic
- 1 tablespoon fresh rosemary, for garnish
- 1 tablespoon black peppercorns
- 1 teaspoon salt

Directions:

1. Preheat the grill. Grease the pan with cooking spray.
2. Meanwhile, in a bowl, combine turkey chunks, garlic, ½ cup rosemary, and peppercorns. Chill for 1 hour.
3. Remove the turkey from the bowl and season with salt.
4. Cook the turkey for 4 minutes. Pour the remaining lemon juice.

5. Serve and garnish with rosemary leaves

33. Grilled Rib Eye

Ingredients:
- 4 rib eye steaks
- 2 Tbsp. olive oil
- 1 tsp. garlic, minced
- 1 tsp. dried rosemary
- 1 tsp. red pepper flakes
- Pinch of sea salt
- 1 tsp. black peppercorns

Directions:
1. Combine olive oil, garlic, rib eye steaks, black peppercorns, dried rosemary, thin lemon medallions, and red pepper flakes. Transfer ingredients in a freezer-safe bag. Seal.
2. Massage vigorously to tenderize the meat. Set aside for 1 hour before grilling.
3. Drain the meat. Discard lemon medallions.
4. Grill the rib eye steaks for 10 minutes if you want it medium rare. Grill for 15 minutes if you want it well-done.
5. Transfer to a plate and cover with aluminum foil. Let the steak cool for 5 minutes. Season with salt.

34. Chicken Kebabs

Ingredients:
- 2 lbs. chicken breasts, boneless and skinless, rinsed thoroughly, blot dried with paper towel
- 3 garlic cloves, crushed
- ¾ cup olive oil
- Pinch of sea salt, to taste
- Pinch of ground black pepper

Directions:

1. Preheat the grill to medium heat.
2. Chop chicken breasts into bite-sized chunks. Set aside.
3. Meanwhile, mix olive oil with garlic. Mix. Season with salt and pepper.
4. Place chicken cubes into the mixture. Toss well to coat.
5. Place inside the fridge, covered for 12 hours to marinate.
6. Once ready to cook, combine olive oil with salt and pepper.
7. Skewer the chicken. Coat kebabs in the lemon and olive oil mixture.
8. Grill for 10 minutes, basting and turning occasionally. Transfer to a serving platter.
9. Allow chicken to cool before serving.

35. Garlic Steaks with Vinegar

Ingredients:
- 2 cups lean beef minute steaks
- 2 tsp. balsamic vinegar
- 2 garlic cloves, chopped finely
- 3 tbsp. olive oil, divided

Directions:
1. Season steak with salt, pepper, and olive oil.
2. Spray oil to the pan. Cook steak for 2 minutes on each side. Transfer steaks to a plate. Set aside.
3. Pour remaining olive oil in a pan. Saute garlic. Cook for 2 minutes. Pour balsamic vinegar. Season with salt and pepper.
4. Divide steaks among microwaveable containers. Put balsamic dressing.
5. This will keep in the fridge for up to 3 days. Reheat before serving.
6. Dish is best served with brown rice.

36. Mexican Chops

Ingredients:
- 2 lbs pork loin, boneless
- 2 garlic cloves, minced
- 1 tbsp. cumin
- 2 tbsp. extra virgin olive oil
- 1 tbsp. cracked black pepper

Side Dish
- 2 garlic cloves, minced
- 1 tbsp. erythritol
- Pinch of salt
- Pinch of ground black pepper
- Olive oil

Directions:
1. Preheat the grill.
2. Mix the cumin, black pepper, salt and olive oil in a bowl. Spread the marinade into the meat. Grill for several minutes on each side. Flip then continue to grill until done.
3. For the side dish, pour olive oil in the pan and place it over medium heat.
4. Cook the garlic until it is fragrant and brown. Mix in the erythritol and seasoning. Cook for another 5 minutes. Serve on the side.

37. Jerk Pork Tenderloin

Ingredients:
- 1 tablespoon jerk seasoning
- 1 lb pork tenderloin
- 2 tablespoons olive oil
- 1 ½ teaspoons curry powder
- 2 tablespoons chopped cilantro
- 1 12/ teaspoons erythritol
- 1 ½ teaspoons ginger, minced

Directions:
1. Preheat the grill over medium-high. Grease the pan with cooking spray.
2. Rub jerk seasoning all over the pork. Drizzle with olive oil.
3. Put on the grill rack. Cook until a thermometer registers 160 degrees F.
4. To make the salsa, put eryhtritol, cilantro, and ginger in a bowl. Toss well to combine.
5. Cut pork into bite size pieces and serve with the salsa.

38. Lamb Chops in Cinnamon Sauce

Ingredients:

For the lamb chops
- ☐ 4 pieces lean lamb chops, bone in
- ☐ 1 tsp. olive oil
- ☐ Pinch of sea salt
- ☐ pinch of pepper, to taste
- ☐ Dash of Spanish paprika

- ☐ 2 tsp. cinnamon powder
- ☐ Dash of cayenne powder
- ☐ 2 Tbsp. erythritol
- ☐ 1 tsp. olive oil
- ☐ 1 tsp. butter
- ☐ ½ cup apple cider vinegar
- ☐ ¼ cup double cream

Directions:
1. For the lamb chops, season lean meat with paprika, salt, and pepper. Cook lamb chops for 5 minutes or until lightly seared.

2. Place meat to a plate lined with aluminum foil. Allow the cooked lamb to rest for 5 minutes.
3. Meanwhile, in a small mixing bowl, erythritol, cinnamon, and cayenne pepper in apple cider vinegar. Stir well. Pour mixture onto the lamb chops into the skillet.
4. Reduce heat and let it simmer for 10 minutes. Tip in heavy cream. Serve.

39. Knaidlach and Chicken Soup

Ingredients :

For the Knaidlach
- ½ cup matzo meal
- 2 eggs
- 2 Tbsp. margarine, melted
- 3 Tbsp. water
- Pinch of kosher salt, add more if needed
- Pinch of ground black pepper, to taste

For the Soup
- 2 lbs. chicken, chopped
- ¾ cup white wine vinegar
- 1 onion, sliced into wedges
- 1 ginger, sliced thinly
- 2 Tbsp. fresh cilantro, chopped
- 2 fresh thyme sprigs
- 1 rosemary sprig
- 2 bay leaves
- 12 black peppercorns
- Pinch of salt, add more if needed

Directions:
1. For the Knaidlach, beat the eggs in a bowl or until frothy. Add in melted margarine. Season with salt and pepper. Stir in parsley. mix well.

2.   Gradually add in matzo meal into the egg mixture. Pour water. Mix the ingredients until pasty. Cover and place inside the fridge for 2 hours or overnight
3.   Once the dough is chilled, line a tray with plastic wrap. Form the dough into and line them up on the tray.
4.   boil salted water in a pot. Once boiling, reduce the heat and add the balls. Cover and allow to simmer for 20 minutes or until tender.
5.   Transfer knaidlach on a baking sheet. Set aside.
6.   For the soup, pour olive oil in a large saucepan. Cook chicken pieces for 8 minutes or until cooked through and browned all over. Darin on paper towels.
7.   Pour white wine vinegar and allow to simmer for 1 minute. Add in cooked chicken pieces. Pour water.
8.   Add in onions into the pot. Put bay leaves, peppercorns, ginger, and salt. Pour just enough water.
9.   Allow the soup to simmer for 1 hour. Before the 1 hour mark, take the chicken pieces out and transfer in a large bowl. Scrape meat off the bones.
10. Discard all solids. return shredded chicken back into the soup together with the knaidlach. Serve.

40. Rack of Lamb in Mint

Ingredients:
- 8-rib rack of lamb
- 1 tablespoon bread crumbs dried
- 1 tablespoon fresh mint, chopped
- 1 garlic clove, minced
- 1 teaspoon olive oil
- ¼ teaspoon salt
- ¼ teaspoon black pepper

Directions:
1. Preheat the grill. Coat with nonstick spray.
2. Rub lamb with salt and pepper all over. Grill for 10 minutes or until browned. Remove from grill and set aside.
3. In a bowl, mix together bread crumbs, olive oil, fresh mint, and garlic. Rub mixture on lamb and spray the crumb mixture with nonstick spray.
4. Put the lamb back on the grill. Grill until an instant-read thermometer registers 145 degrees Fahrenheit.
5. Cover grilled lamb with foil and let sit for 10 minutes. Slice into chops.

41. Herbed Cheese Chicken

Ingredients:
- 4 skinless boneless chicken, halved
- 2 teaspoons tarragon, chopped
- 1 tablespoon parsley, chopped
- 1 tablespoon dill, chopped
- 3 tablespoons basil, chopped
- ½ reduced-fat goat cheese, crumbled
- ½ teaspoon salt
- ¼ teaspoon pepper

Directions:
1. Preheat the grill to medium-high. Coat grill rack with nonstick spray.
2. In a bowl, combine tarragon, parsley, dill, and basil. Add goat cheese into the mixture. Set aside some of the herb mixture.
3. Make a small pocket in the chicken breast. Each pocket should be filled with the herb mixture. Secure pocket using a toothpick. Season with salt, pepper, and herb mixture.
4. Grill chicken for 10 minutes on each side. Serve.

42. Herbed Cheese Chicken Fingers

Ingredients:
- 2 lbs. chicken breast, boneless, skinless, rinsed thoroughly, blot dry with paper towels, slice into fingers
- ½ cup butter
- 2 Tbsp. fresh thyme, chopped
- 4 garlic cloves, chopped
- 1 cup Parmesan cheese, grated
- 1 tsp. chili pepper flakes
- Olive oil
- Pinch of sea salt
- Pinch of ground black pepper, to taste

Directions:
1. Preheat the oven to 350 degrees F. Lightly grease a baking sheet with olive oil. Set aside.
1. Pour butter on the saucepan set over medium heat.
2. Once butter is melted, saute garlic until fragrant. Remove from heat set aside.
3. Meanwhile, put together thyme, chili pepper, and Parmesan cheese. Season with salt and pepper. Stir to combine. Set aside.
4. Coat chicken fingers in garlic butter mixture.
5. Dredge chicken in cheesy mixture. Layer on the baking sheet.
6. Place inside the oven and bake for 30 minutes, or until golden brown and cooked through.
7. Transfer to a cooling rack and let cool completely.
8. For leftovers, store in an airtight container. This will keep in the fridge for up to 3 days. Reheat before serving.

43. Creamy Chicken Soup

Ingredients:
- 1 cup chicken breast, diced, cooked
- Dried herbs de Provence, to taste
- 1 onion, diced

- 2 cups chicken stock
- ¼ cup olive oil
- ½ cup water
- Pinch of sea salt, to taste

Directions:
1. Pour olive oil in a saucepan. Once hot, sauté onion, celery, and carrot, until the onion is translucent.
2. Add in macadamia nuts. Pour chicken stock.
3. Bring mixture to a boil. Once boiling, reduce to a simmer until the carrots are tender.
4. Turn off the heat. Let cool. Blend mixture using an immersion blender until smooth and the nuts pureed. Pour mixture back into the saucepan.
5. Add water into the soup. Stir. Add in chicken.
6. To serve, ladle soup into bowls.
7. For leftovers, store in an airtight container. This will keep in the fridge for up to 3 days. Reheat before serving.

44. Roasted Beef Broth

Ingredients:
- 2½ pounds beef bones
- 1 Tbsp. dried rosemary
- 2 whole dried bay leaves
- 3 Tbsp. balsamic vinegar
- water
- 1 tsp. dried oregano
- Pinch of sea salt, add more if needed
- 1 black peppercorns, cracked

Directions:
1. Preheat the oven to 350°F. Line a roasting tin and a baking sheet with aluminum foil.
2. Layer beef bones in the roasting tin, meat side up. Place the roasting tin on the topmost part of the oven.

3.   Roast for 25 minutes or until browned all over. Flip and then roast other side for another 15 minutes. Remove the tin from the oven.
4.   Place the garlic heads in the corners of the baking sheet. Season with salt. Drizzle in olive oil. Roast for 25 minutes.
5.   For the broth, transfer contents of the baking sheet and the roasting tin into a stockpot. Pour water, vinegar, dried rosemary, bay leaves, oregano, salt, and black peppercorns.
6.   Bring mixture to a rolling boil. Secure the lid. Reduce the heat and allow to simmer for 2 hours. Stir occasionally.
7.   Turn off the heat. Let the broth cool. Discard solids. Adjust taste if needed.
8.   Pour the broth in a freezer-safe container. Place inside the freezer for 2 hours or until ready to serve.

45. Grilled Catfish Fillets

Ingredients:

- 4 pieces catfish fillets
- 2 Tbsp. Spanish paprika powder
- 1 tsp. red pepper flakes
- Pinch of sea salt
- olive oil for brushing

Directions:
1.   For the grill fish, lightly grease the grill pan with olive oil.
2.   In a small mixing bowl, put together paprika and salt. Mix well. Season catfish fillets using this mixture.
3.   Grill for 5 minutes on one side and then flip through the other side and cook for another 4 minutes.
4.   Transfer grilled fillets to a platter and cover with aluminum foil. Allow to rest for 2 minutes.
5.   To serve, place few pieces of fish fillet on a plate.

46. Turkey Sliders

Ingredients:
- 8 dinner rolls
- Light mayonnaise
- Unsweetened mustard

For the Burger
- 1½ pound lean ground turkey
- Pinch of sea salt, add more if needed
- Pinch of white pepper, to taste
- 2 tsp. olive oil, for greasing

Directions:
1. Set the grill pan over medium heat. Lightly grease the cooking surface. With olive oil
2. Put together lean ground turkey, salt, and white pepper in a mixing bowl. Shape into equal sized patties. Grill burgers patties for 5 minutes, flipping once.
3. Transfer the burgers to a plate with aluminum foil. Allow patties to rest for another 5 minutes.
4. To serve, spread mayonnaise on half of the dinner rolls. Place a burger patty on top, spread mustard on the other half of dinner rolls. Seal sliders. Serve.

47. No Salt Beef Stock

Ingredients:
- 2½ pounds beef bones, preferably with marrow and meat
- 2 Tbsp. apple cider vinegar
- 6 cups water
- 1 onion, quartered
- 1 tsp. whole black peppercorns

Directions:

1. Preheat the oven to 350°F. Line a roasting tin with aluminum foil.
2. Layer beef bones in the roasting tin, marrow side up.
3. Roast for 25 minutes or until browned all over. Flip the bones. Roast for another 10 minutes. Remove tin from oven.
4. Transfer contents of roasting tin into a suitable-sized slow cooker.
5. Pour apple cider vinegar, onion, and black peppercorns into the slow cooker. Stir.
6. Secure the lid and lock in place. Cook the broth for 8 hours, undisturbed.
7. Turn off the heat. Allow to cool at room temperature before straining the solids. Adjust taste if needed.
8. Pour the broth in a freezer-safe container. Place inside the freezer for 2 hours or until ready to use.
9. To serve, simply reheat desired amount of broth into a bowl. Place inside the microwave oven.

48. Sweet and Sour Beef Balls

Ingredients:

For the Meatballs
- 2½ pounds lean ground beef
- oil, for greasing
- 1 Tbsp. almond flour, finely milled
- 2 eggs, whisked, discard yolk
- ¼ cup cilantro, minced
- ½ cup chives, minced
- Pinch of sea salt, add more if needed
- Pinch of black pepper, to taste

For the Sauce
- ¼ cup vinegar
- ¼ cup water
- 2 Tbsp. erythritol

- ☐ Pinch of sea salt, add more if needed
- ☐ Pinch of white pepper, to taste

Directions:
1. Preheat the oven to 400°F. Grease bottom of a large saucepan with oil.
2. Put together lean ground beef, almond flour, eggs, cilantro, chives, salt, and pepper in a mixing bowl. Roll mixture into meatballs.
3. Place meatballs into the saucepan. Cook for 5 minutes. Turn off the heat.
4. Add in vinegar, water, erythritol, salt, and white pepper. Pour meatballs.
5. Secure the lid. Place inside the oven and cook for 40 minutes.
6. Remove saucepan from the oven. Allow to cool for 10 more minutes.
7. To serve, ladle meatballs and sauce into a bowl.

49. Steaks and Eggs

Ingredients:
- ½ flank steak
- 2 eggs
- Pinch of sea salt
- Pinch of black pepper, to taste
- 1 tsp. olive oil

Directions:
1. Season flank steak with salt and black pepper.
2. Meanwhile, pour olive oil into a non-stick skillet. Once the skillet is smoky, cook steak for 6 minutes on both sides for rare, 10 minutes on both sides for medium rare, and 15 minutes on both sides for well done. Choose desired doneness.
3. Transfer to a plate and loosen aluminum foil.
4. In the same skillet, crack the eggs. Cook for 3 minutes.

DINNER RECIPES

50. Creamy Halibut Fillets

Ingredients:
- 2 lbs. halibut fillets, cubed
- 1 ginger, crushed
- 1 cup fish stock, unsalted
- 2 cans evaporated milk, divided
- ¼ tsp. black peppercorns
- Pinch of sea salt, add more if needed

Directions:
1. Put together ginger, fish stock, 1 can evaporated milk, salt, and pepper in a large saucepan.
2. Bring mixture to a boil. Reduce the heat and allow to cook until the liquid is reduced by half. Tip in halibut fillets.
3. Reduce the heat and cook fish for 12 minutes. Stir in the last can of evaporated milk. Cook mixture for another 5 minutes.
4. To serve, ladle desired amounts of soup and fish into bowls.

51. Shrimp Salad

Ingredients:
- ½ lb. shrimps
- 1 tsp. olive oil
- 1 tsp. cilantro, minced
- Pinch of sea salt
- Pinch of black pepper, to taste

Directions:
1. Pour olive oil into a skillet. Saute shrimps for 7 minutes or until well-cooked.
2. Season with salt and pepper.
3. To serve, spoon desired amount of salad into plates.

4. Sprinkle cilantro on top. Serve.

52. Tuna Salad

Ingredients:
- 1 can tuna chunk in oil, drained
- 1 onion, minced
- 2 tbsp. unsweetened mustard
- Dash of Spanish paprika
- Pinch of salt, add more if needed
- Pinch of pepper, to taste

Directions:
1. Combine tuna chunks, onion, mustard, salt, pepper, and
2. Spanish paprika in a bowl. Mix well. Adjust taste if needed. Place desired amount of salad into bowls. Serve.

53. Creamy Shrimp Soup

Ingredients:

- 1½ pound tiger prawns, peeled, deveined, reserve prawn heads for soup base
- 4 garlic cloves, peeled, crushed
- 4 cups shrimp stock
- 1 galangal, crushed
- 2 Tbsp. fish sauce
- 1 tsp. erythritol
- 1 can evaporated milk
- 1 lime, freshly juiced, for garnish

Directions:
1. For the soup, put together garlic cloves, shrimp stock, prawn heads and peelings, and galangal in a stockpot.

2.   Bring mixture to a rolling boil. Reduce the heat. Let it simmer for 20 minutes. Turn off the heat. Allow to cool at room temperature. Discard the solids.
3.   Pour 2 cups of the soup base into a large saucepan. Put tiger prawns, fish sauce, and erythritol. Stir mixture well. Bring to a soft boil.
4.   Secure the lid and allow to simmer for 10 minutes or until prawns change in color. Turn off the heat.
5.   Add in lime juice and evaporated milk. Allow residual heat to cook the remaining ingredients. Adjust taste if needed
6.   To serve, ladle an equal amount of soup into bowls.

54. Crab Salad

Ingredients:
- 1 cup crab meat
- Dash of garlic powder
- 1 Tbsp. balsamic vinegar
- ¼ tsp. extra virgin olive oil
- Pinch of sea salt
- Pinch of white pepper, to taste
- 1 Tbsp. chives, minced

Directions:
1.   Combine crab meat, chives, balsamic vinegar, garlic powder, and olive oil into a large bowl. Mix well. Adjust taste if needed.
2.   Spoon equal amount of salad. Serve.

55. Grilled Lamb

Ingredients:
- 8 lamb loin chops

For the marinade

- 3 garlic cloves, peeled, crushed
- 1 tsp. fresh mint, minced
- 1 tsp. unsweetened and carnivore-friendly mustard powder
- 1 tsp. dried rosemary leaves, crumbled
- ¼ cup olive oil
- ½ cup balsamic vinegar
- Pinch of sea salt, add more if needed
- ½ tsp. white pepper

Directions:
1. For the lamb chops, put together garlic cloves, mustard powder, fresh mint, dried rosemary leaves, balsamic vinegar, salt, pepper, and olive oil in a bowl. Mix well. Reserve half for basting.
2. Pour the remaining marinade into a freezer-safe bag. Put together lamb chops. Seal the bag.
3. Massage vigorously to tenderize the lamb meat. Set aside for one hour before grilling.
4. Set the grill pan. Drain the meat. Discard marinade. Grill for 10 minutes. Baste, flip, and grill the other side for 5 minutes.
5. Transfer grilled lamb chops to a platter and cover with aluminum foil. Allow to rest for 3 minutes.
6. To serve, place lamb chops in a plate.

56. Chicken Salad

Ingredients:
- 8 oz chicken breast, boneless, skinless, sliced
- 1 tsp chili powder
- Cooking fat
- Pinch of salt
- Pinch of ground black pepper

For the dressing
- 3 tbsp. almond butter

- ½ garlic clove, minced
- ½ tbsp. raw honey
- 1 tbsp. ground mustard, unsweetened, carnivore-friendly
- 3 tbsp. water
- 1 tbsp. olive oil
- Pinch of salt
- Pinch of ground pepper

Directions:
1. Season the chicken with chili powder, salt and pepper. Make sure to rub the seasonings thoroughly.
2. Pour the cooking oil in a medium pan and place over heat. Cook the chicken in the pan for 10 minutes until brown.
3. Flip it every few minutes to make sure that it is cooked through. Transfer to plate and allow it to cool.
4. Shred the chicken using fork and knife. Mix all of the ingredients in the bowl and use a spoon to mix it. Adjust the seasoning as necessary.
5. Drizzle in dressing before serving.

57. Steak Sandwich

Ingredients:
- ½ pound sirloin steak
- 1 Tbsp. mustard, unsweetened, carnivore-friendly
- olive oil, for frying
- Pinch of sea salt, add more if needed
- Pinch of black pepper, to taste

Directions:
1. For the steak, season sirloin steak with salt and pepper. Wrap tightly in saran wrap. Place inside the fridge for 30 minutes. Drain the meat.
2. Lightly grease a pan with oil.

3. Wait for the oil to become smoky before frying the sirloin steak. Cook for 5 minutes. Flip the other side and cook for another 5 minutes. Turn off the heat.
4. Transfer to a plate. Set aside meat for 10 minutes before carving.
5. To serve, spread the mustard on bread slices. Place sliced steak on one bread slice. Top off with the other bread slice. Serve.

58. Stuffed Turkey

Ingredients:

For the brine

- 1 lb. turkey
- ½ bunch fresh sage
- 1 onion, diced
- 1 garlic head, cut horizontally
- ½ bunch fresh rosemary
- 6 bay leaves
- Water
- Pinch of salt

For the stuffing

- 1 lb ground veal
- Turkey giblets
- 1 cup almond flour
- 2 garlic cloves, minced
- 1 onion, diced
- 1 egg
- ¼ tsp ground clove
- 1 tsp ground cinnamon
- ¼ tsp ground nutmeg
- Pinch of salt
- Pinch of ground black pepper

For the herb crust

- 1 bunch fresh rosemary, finely chopped
- 1 cup ghee
- 1 bunch fresh sage
- Pinch of salt

For the turkey and gravy

- 5 cups chicken stock, divided
- 2 tbsp. tapioca starch
- 4 garlic cloves, smashed
- 1 onion, diced
- 1 cinnamon stick
- 5 bay leaves
- 1 bunch thyme
- Pinch of salt
- Pinch of pepper, to taste

Directions:
1. Combine the brine ingredients in a large container. Mix the turkey and add the water. Season it with salt. Leave it inside the refrigerator for 2 days. Remove the turkey from its marinade and drain.
2. Mix the herb crust ingredients in a separate container and spread the mixture on the chicken. Coat with ghee and herbs as well. Leave the chicken in the refrigerator overnight.
3. Preheat the oven. Adjust the seasoning of the stuffing if desired. Place the veal mixture inside the turkey and make sure to bind the legs together. Add in onion, bay leaves, cinnamon, thyme, onion, salt and pepper.
4. Place the turkey on top then pour the stock over it. Place in the oven and cook for 45 minutes or until it is done. Reduce the heat and allow the meat to cook for another 30 minutes.

5.   Cover the pan and remove from the heat. Remove the stuffing inside. Place in a bowl. Pour the broth in the pan. Mix water and starch together in a small bowl. Whisk to combine then pour into the pan.
6.   Add the tapioca starch with the chicken. Cook the sauce until its thick. Ladle the gravy into small bowls and serve with the turkey.

59. Shrimps and Mussels

Ingredients:
- 12 mussels, debearded
- ¾ shrimp, peeled, deveined
- ½ red onion, minced
- 2 garlic cloves, crushed
- 1/3 cup white wine vinegar
- ½ cup fresh basil, chopped
- ¼ cup fresh oregano, chopped
- Pinch of sea salt
- Pinch of ground black pepper
- 2 Tbsp. olive oil

Directions:
1.   Place a saucepan over medium flame and add 1 tablespoon of olive oil.
2.   Sauté the onion and garlic until tender. Season with salt and pepper to taste. Pour water
3.   Reduce to low flame and cover the pot. Simmer for 10 minutes. Stir in herbs and simmer for 5 minutes, then turn off the heat.
4.   Meanwhile, pour the wine vinegar into a nonreactive pot and add the mussels. Place over high flame nd bring to a boil.
5.   Once boiling, reduce to a simmer and steam the mussels for 7 minutes, or until they open. Discard unopened mussels, then drain.

6. Place a cast iron skillet over high flame and add the remaining olive oil. Cook the shrimp for 2 minutes per side or until cooked through. Add the steamed mussels and sauté to combine. Serve.

60. Lamb Stew

Ingredients:
- 2 ½ lb boneless lamb
- 1 onion, cubed
- 2 tbsp. ginger, minced
- 3 garlic cloves, minced
- ½ tsp ground turmeric
- ¼ tsp cayenne pepper
- ½ tsp ground cumin
- ½ tsp ground cardamom
- 2 cups chicken stock
- 2 tsp kosher salt
- 3 tbsp. olive oil

Directions:
1. Place olive oil, cumin, cayenne, turmeric, salt, and cardamom in a bowl. Mix well until it turns into a paste.
2. Put the lamb into the mixture then toss to coat well. Heat the fat in a large pan over medium heat. Add the lamb and cook until brown. Transfer to a plate and cook the remaining lamb.
3. Add in onion. Cook for another 5 minutes. Stir in the browned bits from the bottom of the pan.
4. Stir the fresh garlic and ginger. Cook for another 5 minutes. Return the lamb to the pot.
5. Pour stock. Boil then reduce the heat. Simmer for 2 hours. Cook until the lamb is tender, stirring occasionally. Season with salt and pepper. Serve.

61. Pork Roast Carnitas

Ingredients:
- 2 kg. shoulder blade pork roast, rinse, pat dry
- 1/2 tbsp. onion powder
- 1 tbsp. smoked paprika
- 3 garlic cloves, minced
- 1 tbsp. dried coriander
- 1 tbsp. dried oregano
- 1 tbsp. cumin
- 1/2 tsp. cayenne
- 1 cup chicken stock
- Pinch of salt
- Pinch of pepper

Directions:
1. Mix all the ingredients except for the stock and citrus juices. Use 1 1/2 teaspoons salt and a teaspoon salt to season the dry rub. Rub the spices on the meat and place in a shallow dish. Marinate overnight.
2. Preheat oven to 250 degrees Fahrenheit. Get the dish with meat and pour chicken stock.
3. Cover and cook in the oven for 5 hours.
4. The meat should be tender enough for it for the meat to shred from its bone by mere poking. Poke with fork to shred and mix.
5. Serve with your favorite Mexican sidings.

62. Miso Shrimp

Ingredients:
- 1 lb. shrimp, deveined, shelled
- 2 tablespoons yellow miso
- 1 tablespoon fresh ginger, grated
- 1 garlic clove, minced
- 2 tablespoons oil
- 1 ½ teaspoon erythritol

- 1/2 cup Mayonnaise
- 1 tablespoon Sambal oelek

Directions:
1. Pre-heat the grill or grill pan. Meanwhile, whisk oil, erythritol, and garlic with miso.
2. Add shrimp into the bowl of whisked ingredients to coat. Thread the scallions and the shrimp on an eight-inch skewer.
3. Grill the shrimp over moderate-high heat. Turn once if cooked through and slightly charred. This will take approximately five minutes.
4. In a separate bowl, whisk the sambal oelek and the mayonnaise as well as the remaining miso. Serve.

63. Spiced Pork – Slow Cooker Recipe

Ingredients:
- 2 lbs. pork meat
- 1/2 onion, chopped
- 1 tsp. ground cloves
- 3 garlic cloves
- 3/4 cup red chile powder
- 1 1/2 tsp. dried oregano
- 1 1/2 tsp. apple cider vinegar
- 3/4 tsp. coriander
- 3/4 tsp. cumin
- 1 tbsp. lime juice
- 1 3/4 cups chicken stock
- Pinch of salt
- Olive oil

Directions:
1. Heat olive oil in a saucepan over medium-low heat. Sauté onions until translucent. Add garlic then sauté for 2 minutes.

2. Add all the remaining ingredients except for pork. Let the mixture simmer for 40 minutes over low heat. Stir occasionally. Set aside to cool. Once cooled, bring the mixture in a food processor to puree. Set aside.
3. Get a casserole dish. Slice stew meat into cubes then place in the dish. Pour chile sauce over meat while sieving. Marinate overnight inside the refrigerator.
4. Place the marinated meat and sauce in a crock-pot and cover with water. Cook in low heat for 5 hours or until meat is tender and can be shredded easily. Serve with rice.

64. Red Wine Vinegar Chicken

Ingredients:
- 2 chicken breasts
- ½ cup red wine vinegar
- 2 chicken thighs
- 3 tbsp. extra virgin olive oil
- 3 garlic cloves, chopped finely
- 2 tbsp. capers, drained
- ¾ cup chicken stock
- 2 tsp fresh oregano leaves, minced
- 1 onion, chopped
- Pinch of salt
- Pinch of pepper, to taste

Directions:
1. Place the olives in a large pan and place it over medium heat. Add the chicken and cook for several minutes. Flip the other side and cook for another 2 minutes. Transfer to plate and set aside.
2. Mix in onions and garlic. Stir and cook until translucent.
3. Pour the wine vinegar and simmer until the liquid is reduced. Combine the capers, oregano, chicken stock, juice, basil, and oregano. Taste and add more seasonings if necessary.

4. Transfer the chicken to the pan and coat with the mixture. Simmer and stir to ensure that the chicken is well coated.
5. Continue to cook for 25 minutes until it is done. Top with the basil before serving.

65. Meat and Cheese Loaf

Ingredients:
- 2 pounds lean ground pork
- 2 cups cheddar cheese, minced
- 4 stalks chives, minced
- 1 onion, minced
- Pinch of sea salt, add more if needed
- Pinch of white ground pepper, to taste

Directions:
1. Put together lean ground pork, onion, chives, and cheddar cheese. Season with salt and pepper. Mix well.
2. Divide into equal portions and spoon onto a sheet of aluminum foil. Roll into a log. Seal the edges. Repeat the same procedure with the remaining meat logs.
3. Place in a steamer and steam for 45 minutes. Allow to cool completely before slicing.
4. To serve, remove meat logs from the aluminum foil. Slice into thick disks.

66. Crab and Shrimp Noodles

Ingredients:
- 2 tablespoons coconut oil
- 1 ½ pounds fresh shrimps, deveined
- 1 pack crabsticks, shredded (will serve as noodles)
- 1 tablespoon fresh ginger, grated
- 1 shallot, minced
- 4 garlic cloves, minced
- 1 tablespoon light soy sauce

- 1 tablespoon oyster sauce
- ½ tablespoon hoisin sauce
- ½ teaspoon erythritol
- ¼ cup pork stock
- Pinch of sea salt

Directions:
1. Pour 1 tablespoon coconut oil into non-stick wok set over medium heat; fry sliced mushrooms until lightly seared on all sides. Transfer to a plate. Pour remaining oil into wok, sauté ginger and shallot until limp and aromatic.
2. Pour pork stock; cook until vegetables are crisp-tender, about 4 minutes. Add in shrimps; stir-fry until shrimps turn coral.
3. Pour remaining ingredients into the wok; stir fry to combine. Turn off heat. Adjust seasoning if needed. Ladle equal portions into plates. Serve.

67. Mixed Seafood Soup

Ingredients:
    1 can whole clams, separate clams from juices
    1 pound fresh little neck clams
    ½ pound squid rings
    ½ pound large shrimps
    ½ pound frozen halibut fish fillets, thawed, cubed
    1 pound green-lipped mussels
    2 Tbsp. olive oil
    2 garlic cloves, minced
    1 tsp. dried oregano
    2 fresh bay leaves, whole
    3 cups fish stock
    1 tbsp. heaping parsley, minced
    Pinch of sea salt, add more if needed
    Pinch of black pepper, to taste

Directions:

1.   Pour olive oil a Dutch oven. Stir-fry garlic until fragrant without burning the garlic.
2.   Add in dried oregano, and bay leaves. Stir continuously to prevent from crusting.
3.   Pour in fish stock and whole clams. Stir the mixture Bring mixture to a boil, uncovered.
4.   Reduce the heat. Allow to simmer for 5 minutes or until the liquid is reduced by half.
5.   Add in shrimp, squid rings, and fish fillets. Secure lid. Let soup simmer for 5 minutes.
6.   Tip in mussels and neck clams. Bring mixture to a boil. Turn off the heat and remove shells that did not open.
7.   Stir in clam meat. Season with salt and pepper. Adjust taste if needed. Serve.

68. Chorizo and Eggs Mix

Ingredients:
- ½ cup chorizo, cooked, crumbled
- ½ tsp lard
- ¼ cup jack cheese, shredded
- 2 eggs, beaten
- 1 green onion, diced
- 2 tbsp. canned green chiles, diced
- One dollop sour cream

Directions:
1.   Using a small pan, heat lard or oil over medium fire.
2.   Pour the beaten eggs into the pan. Constantly stir to make scrambled eggs.
3.   Before the eggs become done, fold in the chiles, chorizo, and onions.
4.   Remove the pan from the heat.
5.   Sprinkle jack cheese on top of the scrambled egg.
6.   Allow the scrambled egg to stay on the warm pan for another two minutes so the cheese will melt and the other ingredients will stay warm.

7. Garnish the scrambled egg with sour cream. Serve.

69. Spicy Relleno

Ingredients:
- 1 lb. ground bison
- 10 eggs
- 6 Poblano peppers
- 1 tsp. coriander
- 1 bunch green onions, chopped
- 1/2 tsp. paprika
- 1 tsp. cayenne pepper
- Pinch of salt
- Pinch of pepper

Directions:
1. Prepare oven by setting it to broil. Line a cookie tray with foil and place all Poblano peppers. Broil for 5 minutes. Turn over to one side and cook for another 5 minutes.
2. Continue this procedure until every side of peppers is broiled and semi charred.
3. Transfer in a glass dish then cover with a zip lock bag. Set aside for 10 to 15 minutes.
4. Put a skillet over medium heat and brown bison meat for 5 minutes. Put half teaspoon each of salt and pepper. Add coriander, cayenne pepper, and paprika on the meat. Stir to season evenly.
5. Preheat oven (375 degrees Fahrenheit). Put all the eggs in a large mixing bowl.
6. Season with salt and pepper. Beat until completely blended. Set aside.
7. Go back to your peppers and uncover. The steam makes the skin softer, which makes skin removal easier. Gently remove peppers' skin. Continue doing the same procedures to the remaining chiles. Set aside.

8.   Stuff pepper with meat mixture then place into a baking dish. Continue stuffing the remaining chiles and line them in the baking dish.
9.   Fill each gap in between peppers with egg mixture. Top with chopped green onions. Bake inside the oven for 35 minutes.
10.   Slice a part with peppers then serve.

70. Shrimps and Chicken Livers

Ingredients:
- ½ pound frozen shrimps, peeled, thawed, drained
- ½ pound chicken livers, thinly sliced
- 1 tablespoon soy sauce
- ¾ cup almond flour, finely milled, add more if needed
- 2 tablespoon cornstarch, dissolved in...
- 1 tablespoon water
- 1 cup chicken stock, low-sodium
- 1 shallot, julienned
- 3 tablespoons oil, divided
- Pinch of sea salt
- Pinch of black pepper

Directions:
1.   Dredge chicken livers in almond flour until well coated. Pour 2 tablespoons of oil into non-stick wok set over medium heat; fry chicken livers until golden brown.
2.   Transfer partially cooked chicken livers to a plate. Stir fry mushrooms in remaining oil until lightly seared; transfer to a plate.
3.   Pour remaining oil into wok; sauté shallots until limp and transparent. Pour in chicken stock; boil. Add in broccoli, chicken livers and mushrooms; cook only until broccoli turn one shade brighter, about 5 minutes.
4.   Except for lime, add in remaining ingredients. Cook until sauce thickens and shrimps turn coral. Turn off heat. Taste; adjust seasoning if needed.

5.   Spoon equal portions into plates; serve with a wedge of lime. Squeeze lime juice over dish just before eating.

71. Sweet and Sour Chicken

Ingredients:
Chicken
- 2 pounds chicken breast fillets
- 1 tablespoon Spanish paprika
- 1 tablespoon onion powder
- 1 tablespoon garlic powder
- Pinch of sea salt
- Pinch of white pepper

Batter
- 1 egg, whisked
- ¼ cup self-rising flour
- 2 cups almond flour, finely milled
- ¼ cup cornstarch
- 1 cup cold water
- ⅛ teaspoon baking powder

Stir-fry
- 1 teaspoon oil
- 2 garlic cloves, minced
- 2 onions, quartered
- Pinch of sea salt

Sauce
-
- 2 tablespoons erythritol
- 1 teaspoon cornstarch, dissolved in 1 cup water
- ½ cup vinegar
- Pinch of sea salt
- Pinch of white pepper

- Olive oil

Directions:
1.   Place chicken ingredients in a food-safe bag. Seal. Massage contents of bag to mix; chill in fridge for at least 30

minutes (or up to 48 hours beforehand.) Drain well the chicken prior to use; discard marinade.

2. Whisk batter ingredients in a bowl until smooth; add more water if flour clumps together, but you need a thick, pancake-like batter for this recipe. Add in chicken; stir until meat is well coated.

3. Half fill deep fryer with oil; set over medium heat. When oil becomes slightly smoky, slide in a few breaded chicken cubes at a time; cook until golden brown. Place cooked meat on platter lined with paper towels. Set aside.

4. Pour coconut oil into non-stick wok set over medium heat. Stir-fry garlic and onions until latter turns transparent. Add in remaining stir-fry ingredients, plus cooked chicken. Cook until limp and aromatic. Remove wok from heat.

5. Mix cornstarch and ¼ cup of water together in a bowl. Pour remaining sauce ingredients in saucepan set over high heat. Bring to boil; reduce heat to lowest setting. Cook partially covered. Pour in cornstarch slurry and lime juice; whisk until sauce thickens. Turn off heat.

6. Off heat, pour sauce into stir-fry when you are ready to serve; toss to combine. Taste; adjust seasoning if needed. Place equal portions into plates; serve.

72. Creamy Shrimp

Ingredients:
- 2 Tbsp. coconut oil
- 2 garlic clove, grated
- 1 onion, minced
- 1 tsp. ginger, grated
- ½ cup shrimp stock
- 2 cans evaporated milk
- 2½ lb. shrimp
- 2 bird's eye chili, halved lengthwise
- 1 tsp. Spanish paprika powder
- Pinch of sea salt
- Pinch of white pepper, to taste

Directions:
1. Pour coconut oil into the Dutch oven.
2. Saute garlic, onions, and ginger for 3 minutes or until limp and aromatic.
3. Pour shrimp stock and evaporated milk. Bring mixture to a rolling boil.
4. Reduce the heat and let it simmer for 20 minutes. Add in shrimp. Cook for 5 minutes or only until the shrimps turn coral.
5. Turn off heat. Stir in bird's eye chili, paprika powder, salt, and pepper. Garnish with cilantro. Serve.

73. Oxtail and Sausages Stew

Ingredients:
For the meat
- 1½ pounds bone-in oxtails, sliced in manageable portions
- ½ pound Italian sausages
- olive oil, only if needed
- 2 Tbsp. water
- 2 Paleo-safe streaky bacon, diced
- 2 garlic cloves, grated
- 1 onion, chopped

For the Stew
- 1 cup beef broth
- 2 Tbsp. apple cider vinegar
- ¼ tsp. erythritol
- red pepper flakes
- Pinch of sea salt
- Pinch of black pepper, to taste
- 1½ Tbsp. dried basil, crumbled
- water, only when needed

Directions:

1.	For the meat, pour water into the skillet. Add in bacon. Cook until the water evaporates and the bacon is crispy. Set aside.
2.	In the same skillet, fry oxtail and sausages for 5 minutes or until browned on all sides. Transfer Place into the slow cooker.
3.	Meanwhile, saute onion and garlic for 3 minutes or until fragrant and translucent. Transfer into the crockpot.
4.	For the stew, pour apple cider vinegar, beef broth, basil, erythritol, pepper flakes, salt, pepper, and water to cover ingredients into the slow cooker. Stir mixture well.
5.	Secure the lid and lock in place. Let the stew cook for 6 hours, undisturbed.
6.	To serve, ladle desired amount into bowls. Garnish with bacon bits on top.

74. Spanish-Style Parmesan Chicken

Ingredients:
- 6 chicken breasts, skinless, boneless.
- 1 egg, beaten
- ¼ tsp cumin
- ½ cup cornmeal
- ¼ tsp salt
- 2 cups chile sauce
- ¼ tsp chile powder
- ¼ lb jack cheese, sliced thinly
- ¼ cup cotija cheese, crumbled
- 1 tsp olive oil

Directions:
1.	Combine the cornmeal with the chile powder, cumin and salt.
2.	Using a large pan, heat oil over medium fire.
3.	Dip each chicken breast into the cornmeal mixture, then into the bowl of egg and back into the cornmeal mix.
4.	Put the coated chicken into the hot oil and brown each side for about five minutes.

5. Place the fried chicken breasts on a baking dish and put the cheese slices on top of the chicken.
6. Then pour the chile sauce on top of the cheese.
7. Bake the chicken breasts inside the oven at 350 degrees Fahrenheit for 20 minutes or until the chicken breasts are thoroughly cooked. If your chicken breasts are thicker, you may have to bake them longer than 20 minutes.
8. Serve the chicken breasts with crumbled cotija cheese toppings.

75. Smothered Pork Chops

Ingredients:
- 4 pork chops, bone-in, 3/4-inch in thickness
- 1 cup chicken stock
- 1/2 cup buttermilk
- 1 cup flour
- 1/4 cup olive oil
- 2 tbsp. garlic powder
- 2 tbsp. onion powder
- 1 tsp. cayenne
- Salt
- pepper

Directions:
1. Place flour in a platter. Mix in dry spices, half-teaspoon black pepper, and a teaspoon salt. Combine ingredients evenly using a fork. Pat meat using paper towels to dry. Dredge meat in the flour and shake off excess breading.
2. Heat oil over medium heat in a sauté pan. Fry pork chops in a single layer in the pan. Brown meat for 3 minutes on each side. Transfer fried meat on a plate.
3. Sprinkle a small amount of seasoned flour on the pan. Mix it with the pan drippings to dissolve.
4. Pour chicken stock and simmer for 5 minutes to form a slightly thick sauce. Add buttermilk to have a creamy gravy.

5. Add fried pork to the gravy and coat them with sauce. Let pork simmer with the gravy for 5 minutes or until pork absorbed some gravy. Season with black pepper and salt. Serve with parsley as garnishing.

76. House-Seasoned Pork Chops

Ingredients:
- 6 pork chops
- 1 cup all-purpose flour
- 6 cups oil
- 1 cup buttermilk
- 2 tsps. house seasoning, see recipe below
- Seasoned salt

House seasoning:
- 1 cup salt
- 1/4 cup each garlic powder
- 1/4 cup black pepper

Directions:
1. Put oil in a heavy bottomed pot and heat up to 350 degrees Fahrenheit.
2. Prepare house seasoning by combining all ingredients. Mix using a fork or shake inside an airtight container. This seasoning will last for six months so long as it's kept in an airtight container.
3. Season both sides of pork chops with a teaspoon of house seasoning and 1/2 teaspoon seasoned salt. Pour buttermilk on the meat ensuring both sides are coated with liquid. Season flour with the remaining house seasoning. Get meat and let excess liquid drip. Dredge over flour until both sides are completely coated. Shake off excess flour.
4. Cook chops in oil in batches, preferably two slices at a time. Fry until golden brown. Take a chop and make a small cut at the thickest area to see if it's done. Adjust cooking time accordingly in frying the remaining chops.

5. Place chops over paper towels to drain excess oil before serving.

77. Slow Cooked Pot Roast

Ingredients:
- 4 lb. beef chuck roast, one whole piece
- 3 cups, beef stock, low-salt
- 1 onion, medium, cut into half-inch wedges
- 3 cloves garlic, crushed
- 1 cup red wine vinegar
- 1/3 cup all-purpose flour, prepare extra for coating
- 3 tbsps. olive oil
- 2 fresh thyme sprigs
- 1/2 tsp. ground allspice
- Kosher salt
- pepper

Directions:
1. Season roast with 1 1/2 teaspoon freshly ground black pepper and 2 1/2 teaspoon salt. Coat with flour and shake off excess.
2. Put a large pan over medium-high heat and heat around 2 tablespoons of oil. Put roast on the pan and sear until all sides are golden brown.
3. Place roast in a 6-quart slow cooker insert together with garlic and onions.
4. Pour the remaining oil and heat on the same pan. Put the tomato paste and mix to blend with oil and becomes brick red in color. Simmer for a minute. Pour wine and vinegar sprinkle flour then whisk to thicken.
5. Pour the stock, 1/2 teaspoon salt, thyme, and several grinds of pepper. Simmer for 4 minutes while whisking until mixture becomes slightly thick. Pour this sauce inside the pot. Seal lid and cook for 8 hours over low heat. Meat should be tender by this time.

6. Take out roast and let it sit for several minutes. Discard thyme. Keep the sauce. Season with pepper and salt.
7. Carve roasted meat against the grain. Serve meat slices on a platter and moisten with a small amount of sauce. Serve with sauce on the side.

SNACKS

78. Dark Chocolate-Coated Bacon

Ingredients:
- 12 bacon slices
- 4 ½ Tbsp. unsweetened dark chocolate
- 1 ½ tsp. liquid stevia
- 2 ¼ Tbsp. oil

Directions:
1. Preheat the oven to 425 degrees F. spread bacon out using iron skewers.
2. Layer on a baking sheet. Place inside the oven and bake for 15 minutes, or until crisp.
3. Transfer bacon to a cooling rack. Let cool completely.
4. Meanwhile, pour coconut oil in a saucepan. Stir in chocolate until melted. Add in stevia. Stir well.
5. Place bacon on a sheet of parchment paper. Coat bacon in the chocolate mixture on both sides.
6. Allow chocolate to dry on the bacon. Transfer bacon to an airtight container. This can keep for 5 days in the fridge.

79. Tuna Balls

Ingredients:
- ¼ cup onion, chopped
- 8 oz pack cream cheese, softened
- 6 oz tuna, flaked

Directions:
1. Blend the cream cheese, onion and tuna in a bowl.
2. Shape it into a ball. Roll it in the remaining pecans then place it in the refrigerator.

80. Ham and Cheese Puffs

Ingredients:
- 6 eggs
- 1 ½ cups cheddar cheese, shredded
- 15 slices deli ham, diced
- 1/3 cup coconut flour
- 1/3 tsp. baking soda
- 1/3 tsp. baking powder
- ¾ cup mayonnaise
- 1/3 cup oil
- Olive oil, for greasing

Directions:
1. Preheat the oven to 350 degrees F. Grease a baking sheet with olive oil. Set aside.
2. Meanwhile, combine eggs, coconut oil, and mayonnaise in a bowl. Set aside.
3. Put together baking powder, baking soda, and coconut flour in a separate bowl.
4. Pour dry ingredients over the wet ingredients. Mix until all ingredients come together.
5. Fold ham and cheddar cheese into the mixture. Set aside.
6. Divide dough into small pieces. Layer on the baking sheet.
7. Place inside the oven and bake for 30 minutes, or until golden brown.
8. Let cool on a cooling rack. Serve.
9. For leftovers, store in an airtight container. This will keep for up to 5 days. Reheat before serving.

81. Chicken Shawarma

Ingredients:
- 2 pounds boneless chicken thighs
- 4 garlic cloves, minced
- 1 teaspoon ginger
- ¼ teaspoon cayenne
- 2 tablespoons ground cumin
- 2 tablespoons ground coriander
- 2 teaspoons turmeric
- 2 teaspoons allspice
- 6 tablespoons olive oil
- 1/8 teaspoon salt
- 1 teaspoon black pepper

Directions:
1. Using a food processor, put together garlic, ginger, cumin, coriander, turmeric, cayenne, allspice, olive oil, salt, and pepper. Process until a paste forms.
2. Rub mixture into the chicken thighs.
3. Secure the lid. Using the Instant Pot Pressure Cooker, press the "pressure" button. Cook for 10 minutes. Remove the chicken. Let cool before serving.

82. Salmon Crostini

Ingredients:
- 2 slices wheat bread, toasted
- 2 garlic cloves, peeled
- 4 smoked salmon slivers
- 2 sprigs fresh chives, minced

- 1 tablespoon capers
- Pinch of sea salt
- Pinch of white pepper

Directions:
1. Preheat the oven toaster. Rub garlic cloves on the toasted bread. Set aside.
2. In a small bowl, combine salmon, capers, salt, and pepper. Adjust seasoning.
3. Spread on bread slices. Place in the oven toaster to warm through. Garnish with chives. Serve.

83. Shepherd's Pie

Ingredients:
- 6 slices bacon
- 1 garlic clove
- 12 oz can corn beef hash
- ¼ cup jalapeno, chopped
- 1 tbsp pepper
- 1 tbsp onion powder
- 1 tbsp paprika
- 1 cup Cheddar cheese, shredded
- ¼ cup green onion, diced
- 6 eggs
- 2 tbsp olive oil
- 1 tbsp salt
- ¼ cup feta

Directions:
1. Place a pan over medium heat and cook the bacon slices until it is crispy. Place on top of paper towel to absorb excess oil. Chop bacon into small pieces.
2. Add more olive oil to the pan then cook the diced green onion and garlic. Whisk the eggs in a bowl. Season it with salt and pepper. Add the crumbled feta and bacon.
3. Add the green onion and garlic to the egg mixture. Stir the ingredients until combined then pour in an 8x8 baking dish. Bake in the oven for 20 minutes at 350 degrees s.

4. Cook onion in the pan. Add the jalapeno. Season the dish with salt and pepper. Sprinkle the onion powder and paprika. Stir until the ingredients are well-combined.
5. Cook the beef in another pan. Remove the eggs from the oven and spread the hash on top. Pour mixture on top and spread evenly. Garnish with the shredded cheese. Place inside the oven and bake for 10 minutes.

Chapter 6 – Sample Workout/Meal Plan

SAMPLE WORKOUT

Earlier on we discussed the combo of intermittent fasting and the carnivore diet producing amazing results for people. We're going to take things a step further by adding a workout program to the bundle for even greater results.
You're going to be engaging in a mix of cardio and compound lifting exercises. The cardio is great for the heart, but the real fat burner is in the lifts, because if done at a high enough intensity, you can often get what is called an afterburn; which simply means you keep burning calories hours after the workout is completed. They are also great for core and strength training.

Keep in mind that you are to do these lifts with the heaviest weight your body weight will allow. Also, for time saving purposes, you want to stick to 4 sets of 6 reps for each exercise, with not more than one minute of rest. Start with a few stretches for 5 minutes, and do light cardio to warm up your body for the workout ahead (includes cycle workouts on ellipticals, stationary bikes, or alternating between a brisk walk and jogging).

Below is a sample workout program to give you an idea of what it would look like for someone who just started on the carnivore diet and is working out at the same time. Based on my experience, 2-3 days a week is more than enough to transform your current physique. If you're really out of shape, you may have to exercise more (4-6 days) to start seeing faster results.

Legs
There really are just two exercises you need for blasting out toned legs, and they are Squats (Back and Front) and Dead lifts. Two others that deserve honorable mention are calf raises and box jumps.

Chest
For this you need just four exercises, and all of them have something to do with a bench. They are the Incline Bench Press, Decline Bench Press, Flat Bench Press and Dumbbell Bench Press.

Back
To develop this compound muscle group, you will need to employ the use of rows. Three of them especially. They are bent over rows, rack pulls, and dumbbell rows.

Arms
You want great looking arms? Simple. You call in the services of the barbell curls, dumbbell curls, and skull crushers.

Core
The core is your center and from where all of your functional strength emanates. Boost this with body weight exercises such as pull-ups, chin-ups, pushups and sit-ups.

Now that you know what to do, here's when to do them.

Monday - Deadlifts, Back squats, Front squats.
Tuesday - Rest – you can still do some gentle stretching or yoga
Wednesday - Bent Over Row, Flat Bench Press, Decline Bench Press, Rack pulls. Core and strength training
Thursday - Dumbbell Rows, Dumbbell Bench, Barbell Curls, Front squats
Friday - Rest day

Saturday - Core and strength training – Incline Bench Press, pull-ups, chin-ups, pushups and sit-ups.

Sunday – Rest.

Working out this hard means your body will be needing vast reserves of fuel, and guess who's now got knowledge of the best diet to meet this demand? You of course.

DIET PLAN

Getting started in your journey towards an all meat diet is extremely simple. Take a look at the sample meal plan below. Basically, you will just have to substitute vegetables and other foodstuff for a more carnivore-friendly meal.
Here's what the carnivore diet looks like:

Breakfast - Bacon and eggs with water or black coffee
Lunch – Chicken, pork, beef, or salmon with water
Dinner - Steak or ribeye with butter
Snack – Chomps or Pork rinds

I was on a 2-week work visit to Nigeria, when I noticed that they had roadside stands with assorted chicken and fish parts just roasting on the grill, next to some peeled plantains. When paired with a simple training regimen, you can bet that that was all I had for the duration of my stay, and I felt great. There is really no need to make things complicated. If you like to eat steak a lot, you can have it for breakfast, lunch, or dinner! And that still counts as carnivore-friendly.

EATING OUT CARNIVORE STYLE (MEAL PLAN)

The best thing about being in a carnivore diet is that there are a growing number of restaurants that cater to an all meat diet. From barbecue to steak, it's not really that hard not to chance upon a restaurant that doesn't serve meat.

All you have to take note of is the way the food is cooked. Do away with meat with heavy sauces and those that are mixed with vegetables.

Unfortunately, Italian and Chinese meat menus are laden with sauces. If you still want these kinds of dishes, you would have to choose meats with less sauce.

7-Day Sample Meal Plan

To get you started, here is a 7-day sample meal plan based on the principles of the carnivore diet:

Day 1

Breakfast - Southern Deviled Eggs
Lunch - Crispy Chicken and Pork Rind in Lettuce Wraps
Dinner - Creamy Halibut Fillets
Snacks - Dark Chocolate-Coated Bacon

Day 2

Breakfast - Mustard Baked Ham
Lunch - Chicken with Yogurt Sauce
Dinner - Shrimp Salad
Snacks - Tuna Balls

Day 3

Breakfast - Breakfast Sausage and Cheese Casserole
Lunch - Turkey Sliders
Dinner - Spanish-Style Parmesan Chicken
Snacks - Chicken Shawarma

Day 4

Breakfast - Sausage Burger Patty
Lunch - Chicken Meatball Soup
Dinner - House-Seasoned Pork Chops
Snacks - Shepherd's Pie

Day 5

Breakfast - Roasted Pork Tacos
Lunch - Steaks and Eggs
Dinner - Grilled Lamb
Snacks - Salmon Crostini

Day 6

Breakfast - Steak Tacos
Lunch - Beef Stew
Dinner - Creamy Shrimp Soup
Snacks - Ham and Cheese Puffs

Day 7

Breakfast - Baked Chicken and Eggs
Lunch – Curried Salmon
Dinner - Tuna Salad
Snacks - Chicken Shawarma

Shopping List

- [ ] Bacon
- [ ] Pork sausages
- [ ] Pork chops
- [ ] Pork belly
- [ ] Lamb Chops
- [ ] Chicken breasts
- [ ] Ground beef
- [ ] Porterhouse steak
- [ ] Ribeye steak
- [ ] beef
- [ ] Salmon cutlets
- [ ] Trout
- [ ] Butter
- [ ] Cheese
- [ ] Chicken breasts
- [ ] Topside of beef
- [ ] Lamb chops
- [ ] Salmon cutlets
- [ ] Ribeye steak
- [ ] Ribeye steak
- [ ] 100% pork sausages
- [ ] Porterhouse steak
- [ ] Pork chops
- [ ] Beef liver
- [ ] Bone Marrow
- [ ] Chicken
- [ ] Organ meat
- [ ] Brain
- [ ] Heart
- [ ] Kidneys
- [ ] Liver
- [ ] Lungs
- [ ] Tongue
- [ ] Turkey
- [ ] Cod

- ☐ Herring
- ☐ Haddock
- ☐ Mackerel
- ☐ Oysters
- ☐ Salmon
- ☐ Shrimp
- ☐ Whitebait
- ☐ Cheese
- ☐ Eggs
- ☐ Heavy cream/full-fat milk
- ☐ Salt
- ☐ Bone broth
- ☐ Unsweetened mustard, carnivore-friendly
- ☐ Non-alcoholic alternatives such as red and white wine vinegar
- ☐ Dark Chocolate – in moderation

Food to Avoid

- ☐ Grains such as pasta, rice, quinoa, wheat, etc.
- ☐ Fruits such as apples, bananas, berries, oranges, kiwi, etc.
- ☐ Vegetables such as cauliflower, broccoli, green beans, potatoes, peppers, etc.
- ☐ Legumes such as lentils, beans, etc.
- ☐ Nuts and seeds such as pumpkin seeds, almonds, pistachios, sunflower seeds, etc.
- ☐ Alcohol such as beer, liquor, wine, etc.
- ☐ Sugars such as maple syrup, brown sugar, etc.

Chapter 7 – Commonly Asked Questions

Question: What are the benefits of following a carnivore diet?

Answer: The benefits vary from person to person. There are people who follow this diet just so they can do away with sugars, while there are those who try to eliminate processed food in their everyday diet. There are also those people who find that an all-meat diet is more beneficial to their health, as it contributes to rapid weight loss, lessened experiences with gastrointestinal disorders, and improved energy and performance among others. Meat is also amazingly filling, so there are lower chances of consuming excess carbs when you feel full on protein all the time. Your body is also forced to burn fat for fuel instead of carbs, leading to a leaner, healthier physique.

Some of the other health benefits noted in the carnivore diet are as follows:

- ✓ appetite control
- ✓ reduced inflammation
- ✓ reduced recovery times
- ✓ reduced joint pain
- ✓ shed stubborn weight fast
- ✓ improved energy
- ✓ improved athletic performance
- ✓ improved mental clarity
- ✓ less eczema and psoriasis
- ✓ improved skin conditions

Question: Does the carnivore diet have the same concept as the keto diet?
Answer: No. It's not the same as the keto diet. Yes, they may both be similar in terms of the concept of limiting some food, but the carnivore diet is essentially stricter than the keto diet. The ketogenic diet allows some vegetables and fruits, nuts, and seeds among others.
In a lot of cases, those who give the carnivore diet a try are those who didn't experience the outcome that they hoped they achieved in the keto diet.

Question: How much is too much protein?
Answer: If you ask 10 different experts, they will surely have 10 different answers to this, but what is clear is that the answer to this varies from person to person. Most people worry about eating too much protein as they believe it may have a tendency to raise insulin levels and blood sugar levels.
However, a lot of research has been conducted in the United States, which proves that the rise of insulin levels is significantly linked to majority of the population following the standard American diet. One which is high in sugar, starch, and carbs.

Question: Is dairy allowed in the carnivore diet?
Answer: This depends on how far you want to go and how serious you are about this diet. There are people who allow dairy in their diet, while there are also those who exclude some dairy due to the sugar levels contained within. So, the decision is all up to you.

Question: Are fruits and vegetable really not allowed?
Answer: As the diet suggests, you are only allowed to eat meat, so you must forego fruits and vegetables. It is a highly debated stance, since a person who only eats meat will be missing out on essential vitamins and minerals that fruits and vegetables give.

However, there are a number of reasons why people who follow the carnivore diet avoid fruits and vegetables.

First, most vegetables are starchy, and fruits are high in sugar. But more importantly, it is the sensitivity and vulnerability of some people to oxalates, antinutrients, and phytates that some legumes and vegetables provide.

But this doesn't necessarily mean that you can't go back to eating fruits and veggies. It just means that when you're starting with the carnivore diet, eating them will defeat the purpose of said diet.

Question: What are the antinutrients contained in fruits and vegetables?

Answer: Plants don't have the ability to protect themselves against predators. This being said, they use barriers such as prickles and thorns or chemical defenses also known as antinutrients.

Animals who are fond of eating plants don't have a way of removing these chemicals. And so, when they have eaten a plant with antinutrients and get an upset stomach, they will be less likely to eat that plant again. In humans, removing antinutrients is done by means of soaking and rinsing.

Question: Who is this diet good for?

Answer: This diet may be advantageous and favorable for those who are looking to change their eating regimen and cut out processed food, carbs, sugars, and all junk food.

This diet may also be good for people who want to rev up their metabolism and reset their appetite for good. This is also beneficial for those who are trying the keto and paleo diet and yet still experience gut complaints and issues.

Question: Why is the carnivore diet still controversial up until now?
Answer: There are two main causes of this diet being always on the hot seat: first, sustainability, and second, is all about ethics.

Both are sensitive topics, so you be the one to decide.

The following things are to be considered before you make a decision:
- ✓ If you are against animal cruelty, this kind of diet is not for you. It's a personal choice.
- ✓ If you are okay with eating meat, you would definitely concur to eat only the best, ethically, and quality raised meat that you can manage to pay for.
- ✓ Consider also vegans who totally oppose the carnivore diet simply because they believe that the healthiest food out there are fruits and vegetables.

Try to think through the points mentioned above and decide for yourself.

Question: Can I be mentally prepared for this diet?
Answer: As with just about any kind of diet, the carnivore diet requires a complete change in lifestyle. Foods that are not carnivore compliant should be removed from your pantry to ensure consistency in your diet. Sounds a bit herculean, but it is what it is.

Whatever you feel about this diet, it is important for you to prepare yourself for the big shift on all aspects – physically, mentally, and emotionally. Personally, the main concern about trying to live on an all meat diet alone, was the challenge of dining in social gatherings. However, the moment you learn to get the hang of it, eating out won't be that of a problem for you.

Take the time to think things over. Do your own research to know more about the diet. Know the pros and cons, and most importantly, know if you can sustain this kind of diet for a long period of time. If it checks out in your favor, do it. Meat heals.

Conclusion

Thanks again for downloading this book.

I hope this book has helped you know the basics about the carnivore diet and the many recipes that you can do with it with the help of different herbs and spices.

If you used to be intimidated by the idea of cooking only animal meat because it seems to be a bit overwhelming for you, now is the perfect time to educate yourself on all things that are related to meat, the best tasting cuts in the market, and the most flavorful ones.

The next step is to try out the recipes in this book and come up with your own meal plan. It would also be best to familiarize yourself with the other meats that you can cook, so you'll never have to do the same recipe all over again. I hope you enjoy re-creating them in your own kitchen, and that you're inspired to pick up recipes you haven't tried before.

www.ingramcontent.com/pod-product-compliance
Lightning Source LLC
Chambersburg PA
CBHW052113110526
44592CB00013B/1589